HOW TO LOSE WEI

In this Series

How to Buy & Run a Shop
How to Choose a Private School
How to Claim State Benefits
How to Do Your Own Advertising
How to Employ & Manage Staff
How to Enjoy Retirement
How to Get a Job Abroad
How to Get That Job
How to Help Your Child at School
How to Keep Business Accounts
How to Live & Work in America
How to Live & Work in Australia
How to Live & Work in Belgium
How to Live & Work in France
How to Lose Weight & Keep Fit
How to Master Business English
How to Master Public Speaking
How to Pass Exams Without Anxiety
How to Plan a Wedding
How to Prepare Your Child for School
How to Raise Business Finance
How to Run a Local Campaign
How to Start a Business from Home
How to Study Abroad
How to Study & Live in Britain
How to Survive at College
How to Survive Divorce
How to Take Care of Your Heart
How to Teach Abroad
How to Use a Library
How to Write for Publication

other titles in preparation

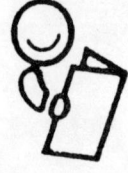

How To Books: General Editor Roland Seymour

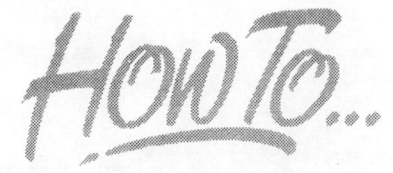

LOSE WEIGHT & KEEP FIT

Aine McCarthy

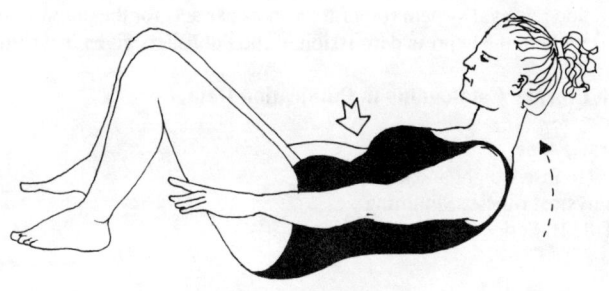

Northcote House

© Copyright 1990 by Aine McCarthy.

First published in 1990 by Northcote House Publishers Ltd,
Plymbridge House, Estover Road, Plymouth PL6 7PZ, United Kingdom.
Tel: Plymouth (0752) 705251. Fax: (0752) 777603. Telex: 45635.

All rights reserved. No part of this Work may be reproduced or stored in an information retrieval system (other than short extracts for the purposes of review) without the express permission of the Publishers given in writing.

British Library Cataloguing in Publication Data

McCarthy, Aine
   How to lose weight and keep fit.
   1. Physical fitness. Slimming
   I. Title II. Series
   613.25

ISBN 0-7463-0571-0

Typeset by Concept, Crayford, Kent.
Printed and bound by BPCC Wheatons Ltd., Exeter.

Contents

	List of illustrations	6
	Preface	7
1	How fit is fit?	9
2	Before you start	25
3	Aerobic fitness	35
4	Building muscular strength and endurance	47
5	Improving flexibility	67
6	Safety and injury	80
7	Mastering your diet and nutrition	91
8	Planning your own fitness programme	107
	Glossary	117
	Useful addresses	121
	Further reading	123
	Index	125

LIST OF ILLUSTRATIONS

1	Muscles and muscle groups	13
2	Health screening questionnaire	15
3	Fitness assessment record chart	19
4	Lifestyle questionnaire	22
5	How to stand	26
6	How to sit	26
7	The pelvic tilt	28
8	Knee over heel	29
9	Side lunges	29
10	Heel raises	30
11	Waist bends	31
12	Waist twists	31
13	Hip abductor lifts	31
14	Calculating your training heart rate (THR)	40
15	Squats	52
16	Leg raises	53
17	Heel raise	52
18	Kneeling kick back	54
19	Side leg lifts	55
20	Lower leg lifts	55
21	Chest press on bench	56
22	Bench flyes	57
23	Arm curl	58
24	Seated tricep press	58
25	Seated shoulder press behind neck	59
26	Upright rowing	60
27	Lateral raises	61
28	Spinal hyperextension	62
29	Abdominal curl-up	63
30	Reverse abdominal curl	63
31	Diagonal crunch	64
32	Gastrocnemius stretch	71
33	Soleus stretch	71
34	Quadriceps stretch	72
35	Hip flexor stretch	72
36	Hamstring stretch	73
37	Gluteal stretch	74
38	Abductor stretch	74
39	Adductor stretch	75
40	Erector spinae (lower back) stretch	75
41	Rectus abdominus stretch	76
42	Erector spinae (upper back) stretch	76
43	Posterior deltoid and trapezius stretch	77
44	Biceps, anterior deltoid and pectoral stretch	77
45	Triceps stretch	78
46	Neck stretch	78
47	Contraindicated exercise: leg sit up	81
48	Contraindicated exercise: double leg raises	82
49	Contraindicated exercise: swinging toe touches	83
50	Essential nutrients	94
51	The food groups	98
52	Example of eating diary	102
53	Your eating diary	105
54	Aerobic exercise chart	111
55	Strength/endurance chart	112
56	Flexibility chart	113

Preface

This book will not help anybody to lose a stone in a week. Neither does it promise a flat tummy in ten days. These aims are usually unrealistic and unattainable, not to mention potentially dangerous.

In contrast, the promises in this book are achievable. It will enable you to devise a healthy, fit lifestyle which is right for you. You will certainly lose a stone and flatten your tummy if you need to, but in a gradual and appropriate way.

The book starts with you as an individual. It looks at your lifestyle, background, likes and dislikes; it analyses your physical condition and takes account of your medical background. It finds out why you want to be fit, and what type of fitness you are looking for. It then brings all this information together and tells you how to devise a personal programme which is right for you as an individual.

It also tries to impart an awareness of how the body works, an awareness which you must have if you wish to exercise in safety.

Because the book stresses adaptation to individual needs, it is addressed to both men and women, of all ages and all levels of fitness.

1
How Fit is Fit?

INCENTIVES TO START

So you want to be slim and fit? Good thinking! People who exercise regularly and eat well look, feel and perform better than those who don't. They usually have well-shaped bodies and erect posture, greater muscular strength and endurance, greater aerobic fitness, and less body fat: the proverbial 'slim, trim and brimful of energy' in fact.

But perhaps even more important is the beneficial effect exercise has on health. People who exercise regularly reduce their chances of developing a number of serious diseases – high blood pressure, coronary heart diseases, obesity, osteoporosis and so on.

Some studies indicate that they are less susceptible to minor illnesses like colds and 'flu, too.

Exercise has psychological benefits, too. Alleviation of stress symptoms, improved self esteem, better body image and a sense of satisfaction are examples.

Exercise also has positive social implications. Now that it's a socially acceptable activity, regular exercisers win the approval, even the admiration, of friends and colleagues. And, unless their chosen activity is solitary, they meet other people, people who are also active and positive, thereby improving their social life.

Summary of benefits
Physical benefits you can gain:

- greater muscular strength and endurance
- increased aerobic capacity (fitter heart and lungs)
- increased mobility
- increased flexibility
- reduced risk of developing a number of diseases
- less body fat, so a slimmer, trimmer appearance

- improved posture
- improved general appearance, skin, hair etc

Psychological benefits you can gain:

- alleviation of stress symptoms
- improved self esteem
- greater sense of well being
- feelings of depression alleviated

Social benefits you can gain:

- contact with other active people
- approval/admiration of others

HOW FIT IS FIT?

The decision to become fit is clearly a sensible one. But what exactly does 'fit' mean? Daley Thompson is fit, but presumably you do not intend to achieve that level. Rudolph Nureyev is fit too, but he could not do what Thompson does or vice versa. A world class weightlifter may be as incapable as you of cycling long distances; champion swimmers usually lack the speed and reaction it takes to be a competitive footballer. This is called the **specificity of training** — in other words, fitness is specific. You become fit for the activity you practise regularly, while fitness for different activities may hardly increase at all.

Another question is the level of fitness you wish to achieve. A sixty-year-old man may consider himself 'fit' if he takes a regular long walk and can do all the things he wants to do. An eighteen year old's expectations are likely to be quite different.

So immediately we run into difficulty when trying to define fitness. It's not as simple as just wanting to 'get fit'. We must consider what we mean by fitness and how fit we wish to be.

One useful approach is to consider the various physical qualities which will improve with regular exercise. We call these **fitness components**.

Fitness components can be divided into two types:

- **Health-related** components which affect the exerciser's health:
  1. Aerobic fitness (also called cardio-respiratory fitness — fitness of the heart and lungs)

2. Muscular strength
3. Muscular endurance
4. Flexibility
5. Body composition (proportion of fat and muscle in the body)

- **Skill-related** components which enable the exerciser to perform activities or movements more efficiently:
6. Agility
7. Balance
8. Co-ordination
9. Speed
10. Power
11. Reaction time

This book is concerned with improving shape and general health through exercise. We will therefore concentrate on the health-related components of fitness. The skill-related components are more the concern of the athlete or sportsperson. So let's look a little more closely at these health-related fitness components.

Aerobic fitness

Cardio-respiratory endurance, CRE, cardiovascular fitness, fitness of the heart and lungs — all these refer to aerobic fitness. The word 'aerobics' came into popular use in the 1980s; it was largely associated with dance exercise classes to music, many of which were not 'aerobic' at all.

'Aerobic' means 'with oxygen'. Working muscles need oxygen to keep going. During aerobic exercise, breathing speeds up and becomes deeper so that more oxygen is taken into the body. The heartbeat speeds up too, to pump that oxygen around the body to the working muscles.

Aerobic exercise is also called **steady-state** exercise: the amount of oxygen taken in by the body is the same as the amount being used. Because of this the activity can be maintained for some time.

A contrasting form of exercise is **anaerobic** exercise, where the muscles get into oxygen debt. Sprinting is a good example. After a few minutes (or seconds) of all-out sprinting, we have to stop. The exercise is *too* intense; we simply cannot take in enough oxygen to meet the requirements of the muscles. We then spend some uncomfortable minutes gasping for breath with a pounding heart, our bodies frantically trying to make up that oxygen debt.

Once we have got to this stage, we are no longer working aerobically, but have moved into the anaerobic phase. The person who is exercising to improve general health and fitness should stick with aerobic work only. All the health benefits which we associate with fitness — reduction in coronary heart disease, management of obesity, lowering of blood pressure — are directly related to aerobic exercise. There is little benefit to be gained from doing anaerobic work.

So what type of exercise is aerobic? Aerobic exercise is any repetitive, rhythmical exercise involving the large muscle groups of the body so that the heart rate is raised into the training zone and maintained there for a continuous minimum of 20 to 30 minutes.

- **Repetitive, rhythmical exercise:** brisk walking, jogging, running, cycling, swimming, rebounding are perfect examples.
- **Large muscle groups:** usually the legs and/or arms.
- **Heart rate:** The rate at which the heart beats per minute. Many things can affect this rate — smoking, passion, excitement and (most importantly for our purposes) exercise. The heart rate is found by taking the pulse. See Chapter 3.
- **Training zone:** the level at which your heart must work to gain all the benefits of aerobic exercise. For example a thirty-year-old man with a resting rate of 60 heartbeats per minute should get his heart rate up to 151 to 177 beats per minute. To calculate your own training zone, see Chapter 3.
- **Continuous minimum** of 20 to 60 minutes: this means 20 to 30 minutes at training heart rate; in other words after the warm up has brought the heart rate into the training zone. Of course, you cannot go out and do a continuous thirty minute jogging session if you have never jogged before. You must work up to this stage. And once you have attained a level of aerobic fitness, you must continue to exercise regularly, otherwise the benefits will decrease.

Muscular strength and endurance

A strong muscle can do more with less effort than a weak muscle. A strong muscle is toned and sleek, not flabby and shapeless. These are the main reasons why people exercise their muscles: size and shape. There are hundreds of muscles in the human body. For our purposes we will be concentrating on the largest muscles and muscle groups.

Working on the strength/endurance of muscle is for everybody who wants a firm, well-toned body, whether male or female. The most effective way of shaping muscle is by using **resistance** which can be increased as the muscle becomes stronger. This usually (but not always) takes the form of weight training.

Muscular strength and muscular endurance are often confused but they actually are two distinct things.

- **Muscular strength** means how much force you can exert in an all out, short-term effort.
- **Muscular endurance** means how many times you can work a particular muscle in a long-term activity at less than maximum effort.

Both qualities are desirable.

Flexibility

Being flexible enables you to stretch, twist and reach with ease. Some people are naturally flexible. Others are less so. But everybody's flexibility can be improved with a regular **stretching** programme. The importance of stretching regularly tends to be overlooked. It is sometimes not considered as important an aspect of fitness as aerobic fitness or muscular strength or endurance. Yet a good stretching programme improves posture, energy and sense of well-being. It eliminates the tightness that tends to invade the body with age. We have all seen old people who are capable of little more than a shuffle of tiny steps as they walk. In many cases the muscles at the back of

Fig 1: Muscles and muscle groups

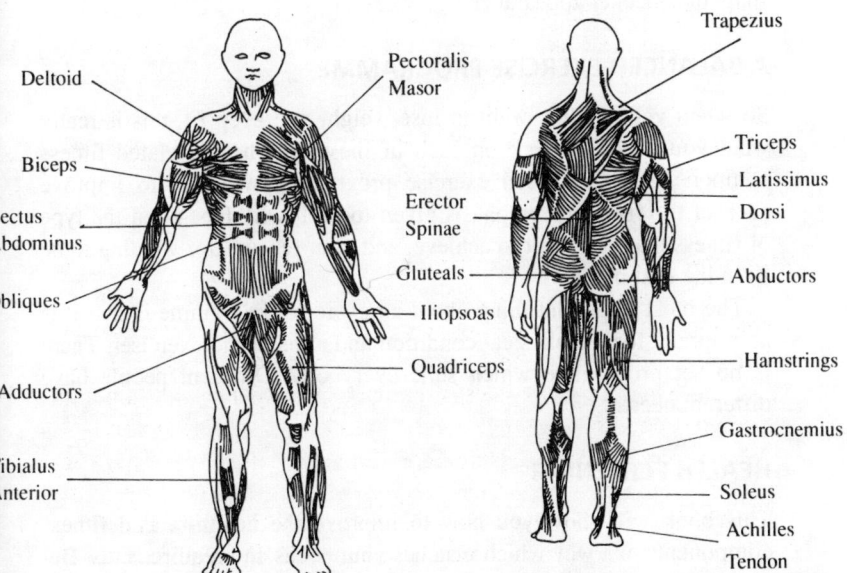

their thighs have become so tight that they can no longer take a full stride.

Stretching to improve flexibility is a very specific technique. The stretch should be held with no movement or bouncing, and no weight or strain on the muscle. The technique is described in detail in Chapter 5.

Stretching is also important for the prevention of injury. A stretchy, flexible muscle is less likely to tear during strenuous activity. Stretching after activity loosens out tight muscles. Therefore a good warm-up and cool-down will always include stretching. See Chapter 2.

Body composition

The reason most people give for deciding to start an exercise programme is 'I want to lose weight'. But weight is a poor indication of shape. Two people can be the same height and the same weight, yet look very different, one flabby and shapeless, the other firm and shapely.

A much more useful measure is the percentage of the body that is fat-free. We all need some fat and women need more than men, but excess body fat is hazardous to health, undermines fitness and is unattractive.

Exercise changes our body composition in two ways. Aerobic exercise uses body fat as a fuel, thus 'burning off' fat. And exercise increases the ratio of muscle to fat in the body, thereby giving a shapelier, sleeker appearance.

A BALANCED EXERCISE PROGRAMME

So when you say you want to lose weight and keep fit, this is really what you need: to work on each of these five health-related fitness components. A balanced exercise programme will aim to improve each of the five. The emphasis given to each will depend on the type of fitness that you want to achieve, and your reasons for wanting to be fit in the first place.

The most important thing about an exercise programme is that it is appropriate for the physical condition and aims of the exerciser. There is no set programme which suits everybody. Different people have different needs.

HEALTH SCREENING

This book will show you how to improve the health-related fitness components in a way which matches your needs and requirements. But

Health screening chart

1. Do you have any of the following illnesses/conditions?
   - Heart disease or circulation problems? _____
   - High blood pressure _____
   - Any metabolic disease eg diabetes _____
   - Any kidney or liver disease _____
   - Any breathing disorders eg asthma _____
   - Any bone/joint disease eg arthritis _____

2. Are you prone to headaches, fainting or dizziness? _____

3. Are you currently on a course of drugs, pills or medication? _____

4. Are you very overweight or underweight? _____

5. Have you had an accident or surgical operation recently? _____

6. Have you ever been troubled by unaccountable chest pain? _____

7. Are you over forty and have you been sedentary for many years? _____

8. Are you pregnant? _____

If you answer Yes to *any* of these questions, you should consult your doctor before commencing exercise.

Fig 2: Health screening questionnaire.

first, it is essential to find out more about your current state of fitness.

In certain circumstances embarking on a fitness programme can be dangerous. The vast majority of people are fit enough to begin a well-designed programme without taking precautions. But there are those who need to consult their GP first, for example those with illnesses like asthma, diabetes, arthritis, and coronary heart disease; women who are or might be pregnant; those who are over 40 years old and who haven't exercised for a long time.

Fill out the health screening questionnaire (fig 2). This will show whether you need to contact your doctor before starting a fitness programme. If you have any doubts, or queries, do make contact. Show the doctor this book and explain your intentions. You will probably receive wholehearted approval.

FITNESS ASSESSMENT

You probably know what benefits you hope to gain from an exercise programme. An improvement in each of the health-related components of fitness is the usual aim, with perhaps an emphasis on one or another. For example a very thin young man may wish to build muscle and strength, a well-rounded woman to alter her body composition by losing body fat, and so on.

Many factors affect what is going on in an individual's body. Health, lifestyle, worries, age, sex, body type — these are just some of a long list of variables that will affect how you respond to exercise.

Therefore, you must form an assessment of your physical condition. It will then be possible to design the programme most suitable for you and most likely to be effective.

Reasons for assessing fitness level

- A fitness assessment will give you a real idea of your present condition. It can be difficult to be truthful to yourself without an objective test.
- An accurate, appropriate and safe exercise programme can be devised for you.
- As you continue through your programme, regular repeated assessments will show you how you're progressing.
- A fitness assessment sets goals for you to aim towards and maintain.
- You can compare your scores with others' if you wish.

FITNESS TESTS

The following fitness tests are very basic. But they are tests that you can do yourself and they will give you a reasonable indication of your condition in each of the health-related components of fitness. (Testing for muscular strength requires the use of expensive equipment, so it is not possible to include a self-assessment test for this component.) Use the assessment record sheet (fig 3 on p.19) to record your score.

After twelve weeks of following the exercise programme outlined in this book, you can take the tests again; you should record a significant improvement. The assessment record sheet allows for repeated assessments every twelve weeks. (Assessing fitness more often than this is a waste of time as any improvement is likely to be too small to be noticeable.)

Cardio-respiratory endurance: the step test

Equipment required. Chair or low table approximately 16" high. (14" if your height is less than 5'3"). A watch or clock with a second hand.

Method
Facing your chair/table, step up with the right foot, then up with the left. Then step back down with the right and down left. Repeat at a moderate steady pace.

(It may help to recite

ON	THE	STEP	OFF	THE	STEP
r.ft.		l.ft.	r.ft.		l.ft.
up		up	down		down

steadily as you go.)

Keep this pace up for five minutes if you can. (If you cannot manage the full time, take note of how long you did manage.)

When you finish, sit down and relax completely for sixty seconds. Now count your pulse for 30 seconds. (Pulse counting technique is described in detail in Chapter 3.)

Scoring

Unable to complete 5 minutes	E
More than 70 beats in 30 seconds	D
45-70 beats in 30 seconds	C
30-45 beats in 30 seconds	B
Fewer than 30 beats in 30 seconds	A

Local muscular endurance: abdominal holds

Equipment required. Large clock/watch with second hand.

Method
Lie on your back, knees bent, lower back into floor. Place your hands on your thighs, arms straight in front of you. Keeping lower back down and without lifting your feet from floor, curl slowly up until your hands touch your knees if you can. Hold this position for 60 seconds maximum. See fig 29 on p. 63.

Scoring

Unable to lift	E
Fewer than 15 seconds	D
15-35 seconds	C
35-60 seconds	B
60 seconds plus	A

Flexibility: sit and reach test

Equipment required. A ruler.

Method
Sit on floor, legs straight, backs of knees down. Gently reach forward, hands outstretched. Use a ruler to measure the distance between your fingertips and toes.

Scoring
2 inches away from toes	2
1 inch away from toes	− 1
Touching toes	0
1 inch past toes, etc	1

Body composition: pinch test

Equipment required. Ruler.

Method
Using your index finger and thumb, see how much flab you can grab from the following sites:
    side of waist
    back of upper arm
    inner thigh
    below shoulder blade

Scoring
A handful	D
More than one inch	C
About an inch	B
Very little	A

Body composition: circumference measurements

Equipment required. Tape measure.

Method
Take measurements at the following sites:
    abdomen – $\frac{1}{2}$" above the umbilicus
    buttocks — the maximum protrusion with heels together
    right thigh — upper thigh, just below buttocks
    right upper arm — midpoint between the shoulder and elbow with straight arm extended in front of the body, palm up
    right calf — area of maximum circumference between knee and ankle.

Fitness assessment record chart

Height _____ Weight _____ Date _____

Cardio-respiratory endurance   Resting heart rate _____
                                 Activity rate _____
                                 Recovery rate _____
                                 Step test score _____

Local muscular endurance   Abdominal hold
                                 score _____

Flexibility   Sit and reach score _____

Body composition   Pinch test score _____
                                 Measurements:
                                   abdomen _____
                                   buttocks _____
                                   thigh _____
                                   calf _____
                                   arm _____

General comments
_____
_____

Fig 3: Fitness assessment record chart

Pay close attention to the precise location of these body sites, ensuring that you always take the measurements at exactly the same site.

Tighten the measuring tape snugly, but not so tightly as to cause skin indentation or pinching. By convention, measurements are taken from the right side of the body.

Scoring

Because of differences in bone structure, muscles size, sex and age groups, there is no fixed set of measurements to aim for. What you are looking for is an improvement between your first assessment and subsequent assessments. In other words, if you are trying to reduce body fat, your measurements should decrease. If you are trying to increase strength and muscle size, your measurements (in the relevant areas) should increase.

A HEALTHY LIFESTYLE

For many people, becoming fitter is just one part of trying to establish a healthier lifestyle. One or more of the following must also be tackled and reduced:

- smoking
- stress levels
- alcoholic drinking

Filling out the lifestyle questionnaire on page 22 should help you to identify areas which might interfere with your wish to be fitter and healthier. Once you are aware of such problems, you can take steps to overcome them.

Smoking

Smoking is the largest avoidable cause of death. Through warning labels and advertisements virtually everyone has been made aware of the dangers, and millions have ceased to smoke. But giving up cigarettes is not easy and there are millions of others who have not been able to quit.

People smoke for many reasons: perhaps because of a nicotine-induced 'high', or unpleasant symptoms when they try to give up; perhaps for social reasons — relying on cigarettes as a crutch to fight nervous feelings; perhaps because the whole ritual of lighting up and smoking is reassuring; or perhaps because it has become a habit, and like all habits, is difficult to break.

Much research has been done on the most effective way to stop smoking. The following three-point plan has proved successful for many:

- **Preparation** During this stage, smokers monitor their current frequency of smoking, noting occasions when smoking is most likely to occur.

- **Cessation** An abrupt end to smoking has been found to be more effective than gradually cutting down. Setting a specific date and making an agreement with another person are techniques which have worked for many others. For example, no cigarette will be smoked by Anna Smith after January 1. If she then breaks this agreement she will be bound to pay £100 to the other party (or do something else which would cause her inconvenience or discomfort.)

- **Maintenance** Stimuli formerly associated with cigarette smoking should be avoided. If after-dinner coffee was a cue to light up, avoid coffee. The preparation stage should help the smoker to identify such situations. Avoiding them may be necessary for many months — perhaps years — until the old associations no longer trigger a desire to smoke.

Stress

Recognition of stress as a human problem is relatively recent, but the physical and mental health implications of a excessive degree of stress are now well documented.

A number of techniques for coping with stress have been developed. One is private speech, where you learn lines to say to yourself before, during and following a stressful situation. For example, before an exam: 'I don't like exams, but I have prepared well, so I should be OK.' During: 'If I stay calm, I will be less likely to have a blank.' And after: 'I did as well as I could because I stayed calm.'

Another technique is relaxation training. In Chapter 5 one relaxation approach — tensing and relaxing specific muscle groups — is described. With practice, a relaxed state can be achieved rapidly in a potentially stressful situation.

Alcohol

Excessive consumption of alcohol causes problems of family disruption, lost time at work, physical and mental illness and death.

There is debate on the most appropriate treatment for those who over-indulge in alcohol. On the one hand are Alcoholics Anonymous and others who feel that alcoholism is a disease and that total abstinence is the only method of control. On the other, there are those who contend that the only thing distinguishing the social drinker from the problem drinker is the amount of alcohol consumed, and that they should strive for controlled, moderate drinking.

Those with long-standing problems associated with alcohol abuse may be more suited to the complete abstinence approach. But younger people who are open to learning new social skills may respond well to the controlled drinking approach. A half pint of beer, single measure of spirits or small glass of wine each represent one 'unit' of alcohol. Men are advised to keep their consumption of alcohol within 21 units per week, and women 14 units per week.

Lifestyle Questionnaire

Age _____

Marital status _____ No of children _____

Do you smoke cigarettes?   Yes/No   _____
If yes, how many   20 plus per day   _____
                                    10–20 per day   _____
                                    5–10 per day   _____
                                    fewer than 5 per day   _____
                                    Occasional smoker   _____

So you drink alcohol?   Yes/No   _____
If yes, how often?   Every day   _____
                                    3–4 days per week   _____
                                    1–2 days per week   _____
                                    Occasionally   _____

What type of drink? _____

On average, how many 'units' of alcohol per night:
                                    1–2   _____
                                    2–5   _____
                                    5–7   _____
                                    8 or more   _____

Do you exercise regularly?   Yes/No   _____
If yes, how often?   Once per week   _____
                                    2–3 times per week   _____
                                    More than 3 times   _____

What form of exercise? _____
_____

Is there any form of exercise that you particularly dislike?
_____

Have you ever had an injury while exercising? _____

If yes, what caused it? _____
_____
_____
_____

Fig 4: Lifestyle questionnaire

Do you work inside/outside the home? _____
Is your work of a sedentary nature?   Yes/No

Which of the following descriptions apply to your job? (Tick as many as are applicable).

Stressful	_____
Monotonous	_____
High-powered	_____
Tense	_____
Enjoyable	_____
Relaxing	_____
Boring	_____
Requires socialising/ entertainment	_____
Irregular hours	_____

Are there factors which limit your availability for exercise?
What are they? _____
_____

Are you aware of the principles of good nutrition?
             Yes/No   _____

Do you try to balance your diet?   Yes/No   _____

What would you describe as your 'food weakness'? _____
_____

Do you find that your lifestyle makes it difficult to follow a regular, healthy eating pattern?
             Yes/No   _____

Are you happy with your
weight/shape   Yes/No   _____
If not, why?   Underweight/overweight

Is there any body area/aspect of fitness that you would like to concentrate on? _____
_____
_____
_____
_____
_____
_____
_____
_____

Fig 4: Lifestyle questionnaire

Exercise, the ideal substitute

In coping with each of these lifestyle problems — smoking, stress, excessive alcohol consumption — substituting positive behaviour for negative can be helpful. Exercise is the ideal substitute behaviour: it makes the exerciser feel positive and healthy, thereby emphasising the negative effects of bad habits like smoking. Exercise has also proved helpful in reducing stress levels.

Changing lifestyle habits can be a long term process but it is often off-putting to consider it so. Set attainable short term goals only, for example not to smoke for one day at a time. If you are serious about tackling a smoking or drinking problem, a number of helpful publications and organisations are recommended in the reading list at the end of this book.

A fit lifestyle

There is no such thing as becoming fit and leaving it at that. An exercise programme must be maintained throughout life. But this need not be as depressing as it sounds. Once you are happy with your shape and fitness level, the new you can be maintained with *less* exercise than it will take to get you there in the first place. In any case, you may find that once exercise and eating properly become a habit, you will keep them up for the pleasure which they give you.

The next four chapters describe in more detail the fitness components which have been briefly discussed here, including warming up and cooling down before and after a workout.

Chapter 6 details the important area of safety in exercise and tells you how to cope with any injuries that may arise during your exercise programme.

As there is little point in exercising without paying attention to what you eat, Chapter 7 deals with nutrition and teaches you how to devise healthy eating habits to fuel your new, fit body effectively without gaining weight.

And finally, Chapter 8 brings all the theory together and, with the help of screening and assessment charts, shows you how to devise your own fitness programme, a programme individually tailor made for *you*.

2
Before You Start

Before beginning the exercises which are going to make you slim and fit, there are a few safety points to consider – posture, and the warm-up and cool-down. These points must be taken into consideration each time you exercise.

Posture is important because if you are standing (or lying or sitting) incorrectly, and you begin to exercise, you will put strain on muscles, ligaments and tendons which are already strained by poor posture. This may lead to injury.

The warm-up and cool-down are important in preventing injury and contributing to the enjoyment of a safe workout.

POSTURE

When we stand tall and correctly aligned, gravity passes through us and we feel light and balanced. But if a part of us is 'offcentre', we bend somewhere else to compensate. This sets up stresses and strains in the body.

Posture is maintained largely unconsciously. Nevertheless it can be much improved with conscious effort by:

- improving muscle tone and muscular strength and endurance
- improving flexibility of muscles and mobility of joints
- concentrating on and practising good posture

You will work on the first two points as you progress through this book. For now, let's focus on consciously trying to improve your posture. Find the nearest full-length mirror, and take all your clothes off. Now stand as you normally do, and look at yourself from all angles.

Looking at yourself in the mirror is essential because, if you have posture faults which have been there for years, poor posture may now feel right to you, and correct posture uncomfortable and strained. Check the following points:

Common standing faults

_____ Does your head point forwards, with chin up?
_____ Is your head tilted to one side?
_____ Does your neck curve forwards, chin drooping down?
_____ Are your shoulders rounded?
_____ Is one shoulder up, one down?
_____ Do you adopt the 'military stance' with shoulders right back and chest pushed forwards?
_____ Is your tummy protruding and your lower back arched?
_____ Is your pelvis swayed forwards?
_____ Do you stand with one bent leg, so that one hip is always higher than the other?
_____ Are your knees (one or both) turning in?
_____ Are your ankles rolling inwards or outwards?

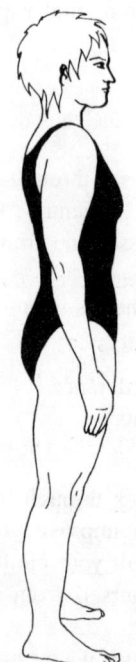

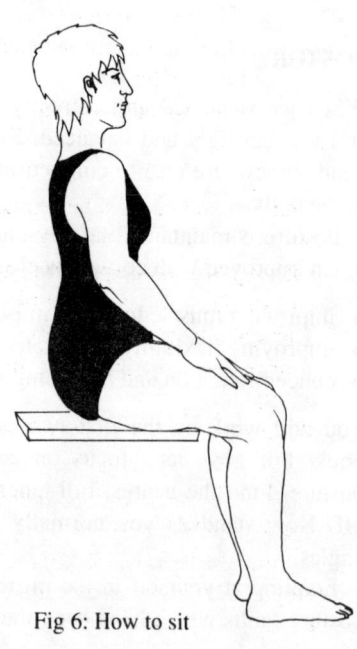

Fig 5: How to stand   Fig 6: How to sit

Before you start

Imagine a string pulling you up through the crown of your head.
1. Your weight should fall evenly through your feet, with the central arch lifted and balanced between your heels and the balls of your feet and your toes.
2. Your knees should be relaxed, neither locked back or bent.
3. Your bottom should be tucked under you, which will centre your pelvis and pull in your tummy.
4. Your ribs should be pulled up high away from your hips.
5. Your shoulders should fall down and into your back, not pulled back.
6. The back of your neck should be long with the chin at a right angle to your neck.

Common sitting faults

Now take a chair, and sit as you normally would, comfortably. Check the following points:

_____ Are you hunched forwards, shoulders up, head poking forward?
_____ Slumped low with no back support?
_____ Tilted to one side?
_____ Legs wound around each other or the legs of the chair?
_____ Legs under you?
_____ Feet turned in or out?

1. Your feet should both be on the floor, slightly forward to relax the calves.
2. Your legs should be parallel and preferably hip width apart.
3. You should be able to feel two sitting bones in your bottom, with your spine lengthening away from your pelvis.
4. Your upper body should be lifted, leaving space between the ribs and the hips.
5. Shoulders should be relaxed, and the back of the neck long.

Posture *is* important. People assume that problems like slipped discs or other back trouble hit out of the blue. In fact such problems are usually the result of stresses and strains which have built up over years, becoming gradually worse and worse, until one day a sudden movement causes something to give way.

The pelvic tilt

Your middle contains two bony structures, the ribs and the pelvis and in between these there is a space which is supported only by muscle. When these muscles are weak and posture poor, the ribs collapse down towards the pelvis. This has the effect of pushing the centre forward in a bulge — a protruding tummy — and of squashing down the discs in the spine.

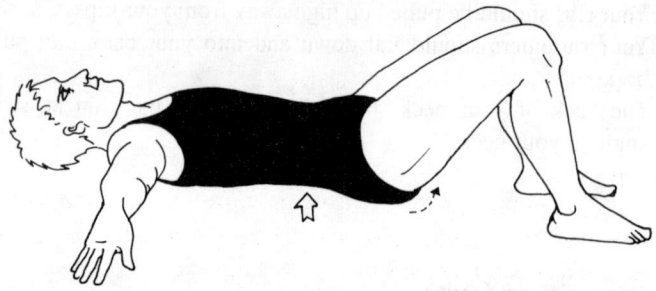

Fig 7: The pelvic tilt

The pelvic tilt (fig 7) can help to realign the body, making the back long and pulling the tummy muscles in. It is one of the simplest, safest and most effective exercises. In a sitting or standing position it can be done anytime, anywhere, without others being aware of it, and it should always be used before starting any other exercises to ensure the body is properly aligned.

Lie on your back and bend your knees up so that your feet are flat on the floor. Contract your tummy muscles, pulling them in so that your back presses into the floor. As the muscles shorten, they will pull the pubic bore forward and up slightly.

Once you can perform the movement correctly in a lying position, you can try it sitting or standing.

Posture checklist before exercising

If your posture is out of alignment exercise will aggravate any stresses that may exist, and you could end up with a serious injury. So before you start any exercise you should ask yourself these questions.

- Am I standing tall?
- Feet hip distance apart?
- Tummy tucked in and bottom tucked under? (pelvic tilt)
- Ribs pulled up?
- Shoulders relaxed and down, back of the neck long?

Before you start

If lying on your side or back, or sitting for an exercise, the same rules apply. Aim for total symmetry to the right and left of your spine. *Check your posture before you begin a workout and regularly throughout.*

The above rules apply to **static posture**, in other words your posture as you stand or sit still. There are various considerations to be observed as you exercise in order to maintain good **dynamic posture**, posture in movement.

As you move through your exercises, stand tall, pulling up the ribs and tucking the tummy and bottom under. Keep the following points in mind.

Knee over heel

In an exercise calling for bent knees, the knee should bend in the direction of the foot with the knee over the heel. Knees and feet going in different directions may put strain on the knee and ankle joints.

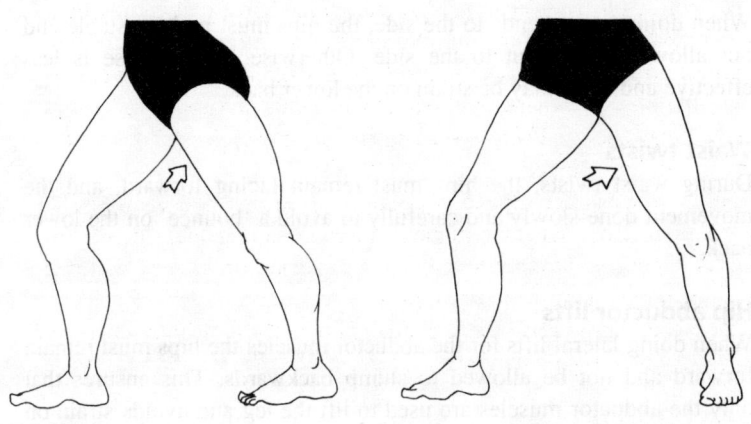

Fig 8: Knee over heel   Fig 9: Side lunges

Side lunges

In the side lunge position, the foot of the straight leg should be flat on the floor to avoid straining the knee.

Heel raises

The weight should be placed over the big toe when doing heel raises. If over the little toe, the ankle joint is strained.

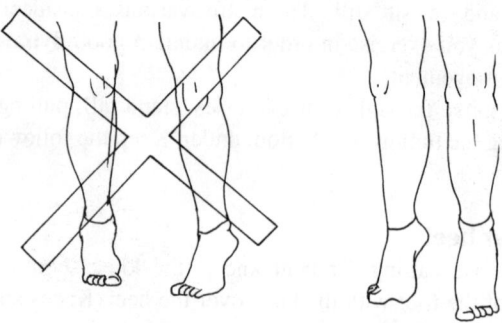

Fig 10: Heel raises

Waist bends

When doing waist bends to the side, the hips must be kept stable and not allowed to jut out to the side. Otherwise, the exercise is less effective and there may be strain on the lower back.

Waist twists

During waist twists, the hips must remain facing forward, and the movement done slowly and carefully to avoid a 'bounce' on the lower back.

Hip abductor lifts

When doing lateral lifts for the abductor muscles the hips must remain forward and not be allowed to slump backwards. This ensures that only the abductor muscles are used to lift the leg and avoids strain on the lower back area.

Locked joints

Joints should never be hyperextended or 'locked'.

Alignment

Any exercise which pulls any body part out of alignment should be avoided. Never force the body beyond its limits. Remember that pain is always a warning sign.

Before you start

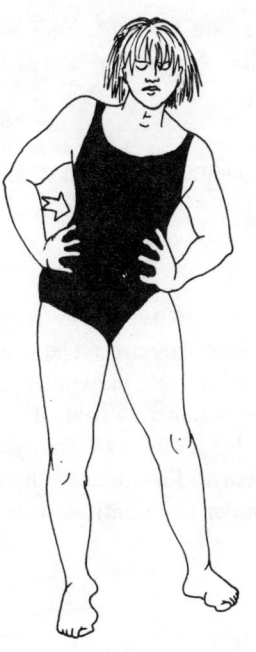

Fig 11: Waist bends

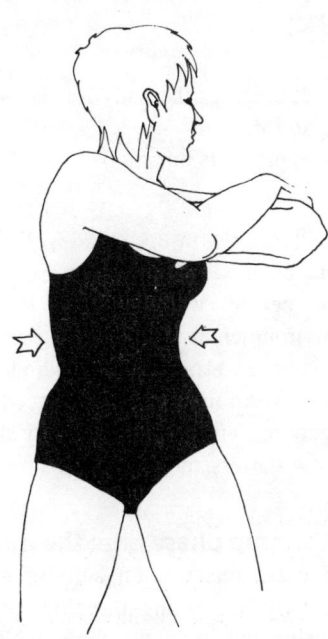

Fig 12: Waist twists

Fig 13: Hip adbuctor lifts

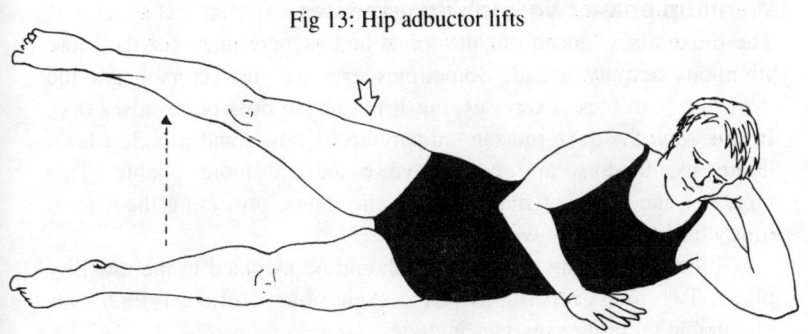

THE WARM-UP

A good warm-up is an essential part of a safe workout. Your body needs time to adapt to the idea of exercise. A warm-up serves two major functions.

- It prepares the body for the endurance/conditioning period which is to follow.
- It prevents injury.

A good warm-up incudes three types of activity: **pulse raising** movements, **mobility** exercises and **stretching** exercises. The warm-up period will vary in length, depending on individual and environmental factors. For example, if the weather is cold, it takes longer to warm up. Those who have acceptable levels of flexibility and who warm up quickly may need to spend only a few minutes on each section. Others — particularly the older and/or more unfit — may be slow starters and need more time.

Warm-up phase one: the pulse raiser

A pulse raiser is an activity which causes the heart to beat more quickly, increasing the flow of blood to the working muscles and raising the body temperature. The activity should be low intensity, allowing the body slowly to accustom itself to activity, for example brisk walking, light jogging, or gentle dance movements.

If warming up for a sport, the warm-up should be specific. For example, tennis players should 'knock up', footballers kick a ball around before play commences. Most sportspeople include this phase of the warm-up but ignore the next two stages.

Warm-up phase two: mobility exercises

These exercises loosen out the joints and prepare them for the more strenuous activity ahead. Sometimes exercise instructors begin the warm-up with these exercises, but it is safer to do a pulse raiser first. In this way, the deep muscle temperature is raised and muscle fibres, ligaments, tendons and connective tissue are more pliable. This increases the range of movement in the joints, protecting them from injury during mobility work.

All the major joints of the body should be included in the mobility phase. Two to six repetitions of the exercise are sufficient. Examples of suitable mobility exercises include:

Before you start

Shoulder	Hands on shoulders, circle elbows. Arm circles.
Neck	Look right, look left. Drop head forward and semi-circle from right shoulder to left.
Elbow	Hands to shoulders, elbows up, straighten and bend arms ('musclemen').
Wrist	Circle wrists. Flex and extend wrists.
Waist	Standing, bend trunk to side.
Middle spine	Standing or on hands and knees, hump and hollow back.
Lower spine	Standing, bent knees, circle pelvis.
Hip	Lift right knee to chest, hold, let go, then lift left knee. Standing lift leg forward, to the side, behind.
Knee	Circle leg below knee. Bend straighten knees.
Ankle	Circle foot. Point/flex foot.

Warm-up phase three: stretching

Lack of flexibility is one of the most frequent causes of poor physical performance as well as a reason for many strains and tear injuries during exercise. During a warm-up it is essential for you to stretch all major muscle groups which you will use during the exercise activity to follow — generally the neck, shoulders, arm and chest muscles, the abdominals, the back and leg muscles.

Chapter 5 deals with flexibility and stretching in detail. Exercises are included there for each part of the body and they are suitable for inclusion in a warm-up.

Stretches are held for just 8 to 10 seconds during the warm-up phase. Ensure that the muscles are warmed by a pulse raiser activity before attempting to stretch.

THE COOL-DOWN

The function of a cool-down is to return the body gradually to the non-exercising state. There are two phases in the cool-down period: **intensity reduction** and **stretching**.

Cool-down phase one: intensity reduction

During exercise, the heart pumps blood faster. And the return of blood to the heart from the lower limbs is helped by the contraction of the muscles as they work.

If you suddenly stop exercising, the heart continues to pump rapidly for some minutes, but because your muscles have stopped working, the limbs, particularly the legs, do not get blood back to the heart as quickly. Blood 'pools' in the legs, depriving other important areas, like the brain, of blood and the oxygen it carries. This can lead to dizziness, even fainting.

The best way to prevent this is gradually to taper off the exercise activity until your heart slows down a little.

Cool-down phase two: stretching

After exercise, particularly repetitive exercise such as running which puts muscles through the same movement many times, you will need to stretch to restore lost flexibility to the muscle. Stretching after exercise also helps to prevent delayed muscle soreness.

Stretching for these reasons is similar to the pre-stretch phase of the warm-up: holding stretches for 8 to 10 seconds.

3
Aerobic Fitness

Cardio-respiratory endurance (CRE), aerobic fitness, fitness of the heart and lungs — all these are different terms for the same thing. For convenience, the most commonly-used term — **aerobic endurance or fitness** — will be used throughout this chapter.

A high level of aerobic fitness is:

- what most people refer to when they say 's/he's so fit'
- what gives your body the ability to jog/walk/cycle etc for long distances
- what helps you to control your weight
- what helps control the development of serious diseases like coronary heart disease, high blood pressure etc

AEROBIC ENDURANCE

Aerobic endurance is not the same thing as muscular endurance. **Muscular endurance** refers to the ability of a particular muscle or muscle group, such as the calves or the abdominals, to sustain exercise for a long time. **Aerobic endurance**, however, refers to the ability of the total body to sustain prolonged rhythmical exercise, reflecting the condition of the heart and lungs (or, more correctly the circulatory and respiratory systems).

If you are very unfit and you take up jogging, it is likely that your heart and lungs — pounding pulse and heaving chest — will stop you in your tracks before the muscular endurance of your legs gives out.

This type of fitness should be the main focus of any conditioning programme as it has a major role to play in the prevention of health problems and the control of obesity, two of the most frequently cited reasons for commencing an exercise programme.

BENEFITS OF AEROBIC FITNESS

Studies show that regular aerobic exercise brings many benefits:

Aerobic exercise and heart disease

Aerobic exercise reduces susceptibility to heart disease. Heart disease (also known as coronary heart disease and cardiovascular disease) is *the* major killer in the western world.

The most dramatic manifestation of heart disease is the **heart attack (coronary)**. Although it happens suddenly, the heart attack is the result of years of atherosclerosis of the coronary arteries. Atherosclerosis occurs when deposits of fat and other materials are laid down on the inner lining of the coronary arteries, the ones which supply blood to the heart muscle.

As the inner lining of the coronary artery becomes thickened by these deposits the area through which the blood can flow is narrowed, making it difficult to meet the demands of the heart when it is under stress, such as during exercise. Eventually the artery can become completely blocked. A blockage can also occur if a clot is carried to a narrowing part of a coronary artery, or formed there.

When a coronary artery is blocked in this way, the position of the heart muscle that was supplied by the artery is deprived of nutrients and oxygen, and dies; this is what we commonly refer to as heart attack. The greater the area supplied by an artery, the larger the area of heart muscle that dies and the more severe the resulting attack.

Atherosclerosis is a long and slow process and aerobic exercise is believed to play an important role in the protection of the body from its effects.

Aerobic exercise and blood pressure

High blood pressure (**hypertension**) is a silent disease which has no warning symptoms. Many of those who suffer from the disease are unaware of its presence. Yet it can kill.

The best control of high blood pressure is through a combination of diet, restriction of salt intake, weight reduction and exercise. Studies show that the blood pressure of hypertensive individuals can be lowered towards normal levels with aerobic exercise.

Aerobic exercise reduces body fat levels

Overweight is defined as exceeding desirable weight values calculated with reference to sex, height and frame size. But such tables are unsatisfactory. Many individuals who are overweight on the basis of these tables have normal, or lower than normal, amounts of body fat. They are slim, fit and healthy, yet these tables classify them as overweight.

Muscle is heavier than fat. So athletes — the fittest and slimmest of people — often find themselves in the 'overweight' category because of their large muscle mass, heavy bones and small amount of body fat. Conversely, many people of 'normal' weight are obese, with little lean meat and lots of fat on their bodies.

So body composition is a more accurate measure of a fat problem than weight. Obesity has many origins: heredity, early overeating, social factors, psychological factors and physical inactivity. Occasionally it can be due to hormonal factors or rare syndromes. Of these factors, physical inactivity appears to be one of the most critical. Much research has been done into the relationship between body fat and physical activity and the following findings have emerged.

1. Physical activity expends calories.
2. Without exercise, the body seems to lose the ability to regulate the appetite and extra, unneeded calories are consumed.
3. There is a theory that aerobic exercise releases substances in the body which helps to depress appetite.
4. Another theory claims that aerobic exercise increases the metabolic rate, the rate at which the body burns calories.

These theories are subject to ongoing research but individual testimony bears out that most people who adopt an aerobic exercise regime firm up and lose some weight while continuing to enjoy their food.

Body fat percentage is determined with the use of **hydrostatic weighing** technique in the laboratory, or by using **skin fold calipers**. But you can get a rough valuation of your own body fat level by using the methods outlined in Chapter 1.

Aerobic exercise reduces depression and anxiety

A low level of physical fitness is frequently found in individuals who suffer from conditions like depression and anxiety. And a growing body of knowledge is pointing to the importance of aerobic exercise in the treatment of these and other mental disorders.

It is also a common finding that an appropriate amount of aerobic exercise makes most people feel better — more energetic, brighter, more alive.

Aerobic exercise reduces risk of bone disease

Bone deteriorates with age and the most distressing diseases caused by this deterioration are **osteoarthritis and osteoporosis**. Osteoarthritis is a degeneration of the soft bone in the joints while osteoporosis is characterised by insufficient production of bone or by serious reduction in bone calcium content. Both conditions are particularly common in women after the menopause, but persons of all ages and both sexes may suffer.

Aerobic exercise has been shown to provide alterations in bone metabolism which would appear to slow down this progressive deterioration.

Other advantages of aerobic exercise

Aerobic exercise has a number of other benefits to offer. It improves blood circulation. Sleep patterns improve and energy levels are boosted. Many report increased self-confidence and a better sex life. There is also the benefit of being alone or sociable, whichever is your personal preference, away from pressures of job and family.

So while aerobic exercise does not guarantee a longer life, it does improve the quality of that life. All these benefits are to be gained from just two or three hours effort per week. No wonder people are catching on.

WHAT IS AEROBIC EXERCISE?

Any exercise which is repetitive and rhythmical, which uses the large muscle groups of the body, and which can be maintained for a continuous twenty to thirty minutes is aerobic. Excellent examples are brisk walking, jogging, running, swimming, cycling and dancing.

EXERCISE INTENSITY

One of the questions most often asked is 'How hard must I work out to achieve all the benefits of exercise?' This relates to **exercise intensity**. Exercise which is too intense is counterproductive. This is the typical approach of the person who has not exercised for years. They remember the level of exercise which they enjoyed when they were young and fit and they try to start back at that level. The result is exhaustion or injury.

So overdoing it is clearly not a good idea. But most of the benefits outlined above will not accrue unless exercise takes place at a high enough intensity. So how do you determine what that intensity ought to be?

Heart rate

The key is monitoring your heart or **pulse rate**. To do this you find your pulse at the carotoid artery just below the jaw bone. Use the middle fingers of your right hand and search around until you find it. It is easier to find if you stretch your neck out. Do not press hard.

Once you have located the pulse, practise counting the beats. When you are familiar with finding and counting, you are ready to monitor your pulse rate. Use a watch or clock with a second hand and time your pulse for 15 seconds. Count the first beat as zero. You should get a figure somewhere between about 12 and 22. Multiply by four to find out the number of times your heart beats per minute.

Your heart rate will be affected by a number of different factors — recent activity, illness, smoking, tension, excitement, alcohol and many others. Practise taking your pulse regularly throughout the day and see how it varies.

Resting heart rate (RHR)

It's best to take your RHR first thing in the morning before you get out of bed. The average rate is 72 beats per minute. Resting heart rate decreases with training so you should notice it coming down over the weeks of following a training programme. A low resting heart rate can therefore be a sign of physical fitness but it is possible for an untrained person, or even somebody with a heart condition, to have a low resting pulse rate.

Maximum heart rate (MHR)

The most accurate way of determining MHR is to perform an exercise test on the treadmill or cycle ergometer to the point of exhaustion. Most of us will not have access to such a facility but MHR can be estimated by subtracting your age from 220:

$$\text{Maximum heart rate} = 220 - \text{your age}$$

Training heart rate (THR)

As you exercise, your heart rate speeds up. By exercising at an intensity that raises your heart rate to a certain level, you can make sure that you are exercising 'aerobically', in other words, that you are working hard enough — but not too hard — to get all the benefits outlined. This level is called your training heart rate (THR) and is a percentage of your maximum heart rate (MHR).

Use fig 14 to calculate what your THR should be. If you are middle aged, obese or very unfit, a THR of 60% of maximum should be sufficient. As your fitness level progresses you can aim for 70% to 80% of your maximum but you should never train above 85% of maximum.

For example, an unfit thirty year old would train at 60% of MHR, (220-30) x 0.60 = approximately 114 beats per minute.

Once you have determined what your THR should be, you are ready to monitor exercise intensity. A few minutes into your aerobic activity, check your heart rate. During exercise it is most convenient to take your pulse for 6 seconds and multiply by 10 to get the number of beats per minute. Remember to count the first beat as zero.

If your check shows that you are above your THR, slow down. If you haven't reached THR yet, increase intensity. After some weeks of monitoring your pulse, you will learn to read your body and stay close to THR with only occasional monitoring.

It should be noted that THR is strictly an estimate. Always be aware of other signs that exercise activity is too intense, such as severe breathlessness, dizziness, and pain in the chest.

Fit
THR = MHR x 0.80 = (220 − age) x 0.80

Unfit
THR = MHR x 0.60 = (220 − age) x 0.60

For example, at thirty years:

Fit			*Unfit*		
THR =	(220 − 30)	x 0.80	THR =	(220 − 30)	x 0.60
=	190	x 0.80	=	190	x 0.60
=	152 beats per minute		=	114 beats per minute	

Fig 14: Calculating your training heart rate (THR)

Recovery rate

Once exercise ceases, the heart rate begins to return to resting values. The speed at which it returns will depend primarily on the intensity of exercise, but also on your level of aerobic fitness. A quick recovery generally reflects a fit cardiovascular system. This is the basis of the step test in Chapter 1.

Aerobic fitness

How long and how often?

We now know at what intensity aerobic exercise should be carried out. Two other questions are equally important. How long should the exercise last? And how often should it be done?

Most experts recommend exercising for at least twenty continuous minutes at THR (aerobic exercise must be continuous, not a stop-start activity). This is obviously a level of exercise which cannot be adopted overnight. It must be worked up to.

Remember too that a twenty-minute aerobic session means exercising for a continuous thirty to forty minutes: five to ten minutes to warm up and get up to THR; five to ten minutes to cool down and stretch afterwards.

With regard to frequency, three or four times a week with a rest day in between is most frequently recommended as being safest and most effective.

USING RUNNING AS AN EXAMPLE

One of the most popular forms of aerobic exercise is jogging or running. Over the last decade, worldwide interest in this form of exercise has taken off, and there are hundreds of short and long races organised for the fitness runner throughout the year.

Running is cheap. The only necessary expense is a good pair of running shoes. It is effective, one of the *most* effective forms of aerobic exercise. It gets the exerciser out into the fresh air. It is an individual activity so you don't need to rely on a partner or team to train with you. Running can be done any time, almost anywhere. It requires no special equipment. It takes up less time than most other training activities.

Getting started

Before you even think about running, you must be capable of walking two or three miles at a brisk pace with ease, and you should also be walking quite a bit on a daily basis. If you are totally sedentary therefore, don't start running; start to walk. Incorporate as much walking as possible into your daily routine: walk to the shops, get off the bus a few stops before your destination, walk the kids to school or walk to the local in the evening. In addition to this, get into the habit of going for a brisk 30 minute walk four or five times per week. Once you can cover a brisk three miles with ease, you are ready to start jogging.

The golden rule at this stage is to take it easy. Begin by interspersing the walk with short twenty or thirty metre stretches of easy running. These stretches need last only a few seconds at first and should only be repeated as often as comfortable. As time goes on, you can extend your jog periods until eventually you can jog continuously for twenty minutes.

The importance of taking things easy, particularly in the early stages, cannot be overemphasised. The price of over-enthusiastic effort will almost certainly be injury. You are making new demands on your heart and muscles and the last thing you want to do is excessively strain either of them. Listen to your body and don't overdo it.

Set yourself *achievable* targets and work *slowly* towards them. For example, aim to include ten short jogs in the twenty minutes. If you can only manage one or two at first, aim for three, then four, and so on.

It may take many weeks before you can include ten runs in the twenty minute period and many more before you can jog continuously for that amount of time. But take it easy. Slow, continuous progress is the surest way to get you there in the end.

Make it regular
Taking it easy does not mean skipping your walk or run whenever you don't feel like going out. If you do this, you will never progress. You will probably find, like most runners, that there are days when the last thing you feel like doing is going out for a jog. The only way to cope with this feeling is to force yourself out of the door. Once you get started, you will be thrilled that you did.

Running *must* be regular if results are to be noticeable, so the most important thing in the first few months is to develop the habit of going out regularly. Make yourself a plan and stick to it.

Some people find it a help always to run at the same time, on the same days, so that it becomes a definite routine. Others prefer to vary their running to fit in with a changing schedule. Find what suits you best, but **stick to it**.

What to wear when running
The only essential item for the runner is a pair of good running shoes. Those forced to do most of their running on roads need to be particularly careful. Concrete is a hard surface with little or no 'give'. Every time you land, a force equivalent to three times your body weight comes down on your foot. If your shoes don't absorb the shock, stresses and strains build up which will eventually be felt not only in your feet, but in your calves, knees, hips and even your back.

Aerobic fitness

Go to a reputable sports shop and buy a good brand name. Try the shoes on, lace them up, walk round in them. Explain the type of running you will be doing to the assistant, for example jogging, racing and so on.

Remember, the function of running shoes is to support the foot. Heels should fit snugly allowing no sideways movement. Your foot should not be wider than the base, causing the uppers to bulge. There should be no friction points, as any discomfort felt in the shop will be greatly magnified when you run. Good **cushioning** and good **stability** are the points to look for.

Break new shoes in gently, walking them around for a few days before you run in them. Never, never wear new shoes in a race. Once you find a pair of shoes that suits you, stick with them, making sure to replace them as soon as they start to wear down.

The rest of your clothing is up to you. Track suits for winter and T-shirts and shorts for summer are the usual choices. But any clothes which allow you freedom of movement, keep you cool in warm weather and warm in the cold, are suitable. If you must economise, this is where you make your savings, not on your shoes.

For female runners, a good supportive bra is essential, particularly for those with large breasts.

Warm-up and cool-down for runners

The importance of warming up and cooling down has been discussed in detail in Chapter 2; the runner who neglects either generally suffers an injury sooner or later. The muscles used in running go through a relatively small range of movement, and this small action is repeated thousands of times in even a short run. This causes the muscles to tighten, particularly the hamstring and calf muscles in the back of the legs.

A stretching session before and after a run helps to counteract this effect, reducing the likelihood of strains or tears in muscles and tendons. It also helps to eliminate stiffness and fatigue.

The muscles most used in running are the leg muscles, so it is most important to stretch these. Sometimes tension or poor posture can lead to tightness in the upper body during a run, so it's a good idea to stretch these muscles also.

The following is an appropriate warm-up and cool-down for a running session. The stretching exercises are described in detail will illustration in Chapter 5.

Warm-up
1. **Pulse raiser**. Brisk walking/light jogging for five minutes or so (more if the weather is very cold) to raise body temperature and increase blood flow to the working muscles.
2. **Mobility exercises**. Loosening the joints of the body. Head circles, shoulder rolls, arm swings, waist bends and twists, leg lifts and swings. Pelvic circles. Knee bends. Ankle twists (see Chapter 5).
3. **Stretching exercises**. To lengthen the muscles and prepare them for activity. Leg stretches are most important but include upper body stretches too. See Chapter 5 for relevant stretches. Hold each stretch for 8 to 10 seconds.

Cool-down
1. **Gently taper off** run to a slow jog, then to walking briskly and eventually to normal pace allowing the heart beat slowly to come down, thus preventing 'pooling' of blood in the legs.
2. **Mobility exercises** as above to loosen out joints again.
3. **Stretching** as above to bring muscles back to their original length.

If you are interested in developing flexibility, after a run is an excellent time to work on this important aspect of fitness. Developing flexibility is discussed in detail in Chapter 5.

Training systems

Unless you are interested in racing, you need never introduce training systems into your running schedule. But many people find that once they have been running for some time, they want to run faster or they develop an interest in possible variations in training. Without increasing the amount of time spent on your running, by including training systems you can improve your aerobic capacity and your running speed as well as add variety.

The following discussion of training systems is largely orientated towards running but the principles are equally effective when applied to other forms of aerobic exercise like bicycling or swimming.

Interval training

Interval training involves inserting rest intervals or intervals of reduced activity (relief intervals) between work of higher intensity. Such a system is usually timed on a running track, and is the most scientific of training systems.

A typical interval training session might include eight 400 metre runs at a pace of 70 seconds with 60 seconds of light jogging as the

Aerobic fitness

relief interval. Interval training can be progressed or made more difficult by:

- making the rest/relief intervals shorter
- making the work intervals more intense
- making the work intervals longer
- increasing the number of work intervals

Fartlek training

Fartlek is a Swedish word meaning 'speed play' and is used of unstructured interval training. In other words, speed is varied but the length of the work intervals and relief intervals depends on you. You can speed up, slow down, run up hills, run on varied terrain, anything that feels right to your body.

This is a free form of training where distance and time are not important; the main goals are fun and enjoyment. Fartlek is extremely enjoyable, particularly if you can find suitable countryside or parkland with a variety of hills. It was originally practised in the forests of Sweden.

Other forms of aerobic exercise

Running is not the only form of aerobic exercise. Other activities like cycling, swimming, circuit training and exercise to music are also popular choices.

All the principles outlined above in relation to running — keeping your pulse within the training rate, maintaining the activity for a minimum of twenty minutes, training at least three times per week — must also be applied to your chosen activity.

So if you want to swim, you must work up to the stage of being able to swim for twenty to thirty minutes before you can consider yourself to be exercising aerobically. Getting into the pool and splashing around, stopping and starting as so many people do, is not going to improve your aerobic fitness.

Choosing an exercise class

If your chosen form of exercise is a class of some sort — aerobics, circuit training, exercise to music, beware. The same criteria must apply. Many so-called aerobics classes are not aerobic at all.

There has been great concern in recent years about the proliferation of unqualified exercise teachers. So do not assume that teacher always knows best. During your first visit to a class, observe closely how things are done. Safety and effectiveness should always be the prime concerns. Use the checklist below. If you see anything that worries you, do not go back to that class. You have only one body — don't take chances with it.

A good teacher
- A good teacher is lively and enthusiastic, and knows how to motivate the class.
- S/he should identify any beginners, introduce him/herself and explain the aims and purposes of the class at the outset.
- Before starting, s/he should enquire whether any member of the class has an injury or illness, and check that they are all wearing suitable clothing and footwear.
- As the class progresses, s/he should constantly monitor the members, checking that each individual is doing the exercise correctly and offering adaptations of the exercise if somebody is in difficulties.
- S/he should be aware of the different levels in her class and offer different forms of an exercise for beginners and advanced people.
- S/he should constantly remind the class about posture and technique.
- S/he should make him/herself available at the end of the class for questions and explanations.
- S/he should have a fit and professional appearance.

The class
- There should be no more than twenty members per instructor. Even the best of teachers are incapable of monitoring more than that.
- People who arrive late and miss the warm up should not be allowed to join the class.

The premises
- The premises should be bright, clean and airy, with adequate ventilation.
- The floor should be wooden and well-sprung, not concrete (or carpet over concrete), which is very stressful to bones and joints.
- There should be plenty of space for each class member.

4
Building Muscular Strength and Endurance

WHAT ARE MUSCLES?

Your ability to exercise, indeed to move at all, is determined by the type, strength and bulk of your muscles. There are three types of muscle:

- **Cardiac** — the muscle of the heart.
- **Involuntary** — muscles which are not controlled by the will, such as the muscles of the digestive system.
- **Voluntary** — muscles which are controlled by the will and which cause movement. They are also known as skeletal, striated or striped muscle. This is the type of muscle with which we are concerned in this chapter.

There are some 650 muscles in the human body, making up 35% to 40% of body weight. Muscles bring about movement through being attached to bones.

Why exercise muscles?

A strong muscle is well defined rather than flabby, and well defined muscles mean a shapely body. Muscle training is for everybody who wants to improve their shape, not just for body builders.

Muscles need to be kept in constant use if they are not to lose their shape and strength. When not used they become weak and flabby, but (thankfully) do not lose their ability to grow strong and shapely if exercised again.

When a heavier than normal demand is placed upon muscles, they are stimulated into growing stronger. As long as that demand remains constant, strength level remains constant. But if the resistance is increased slightly, then the muscle again increases in strength. This is the basis of a **resistance training programme** — to keep demanding a little more from the muscles so that strength or endurance is increased.

The most popular form of resistance training is weight training. But various other forms of resistance can be used. When we do floor exercises without weight, for example, we are using gravity as resistance. Some exercise classes take place in a swimming pool, using the resistance of the water. Others use rubber bands.

Types of muscular contraction

It is possible to exercise muscles in different ways, to have different types of muscular contraction. **Isometric exercise** involves a 'static' contraction, with no movement of body parts. Muscle length does not change. An example is to clasp your hands in front of your chest and push hard, one against the other. Although nothing is moving, you will feel the chest muscles (pectorals) contract isometrically.

Isometric exercise requires little time, energy, space or equipment and at one time was a popular form of resistance training. However, it is now accepted that it has a number of limitations:

- It increases strength only in the position performed and not throughout the full range of movement.
- It is impossible to monitor progress as no feedback is received. It is therefore difficult to remain motivated.
- It can produce muscle strain if prolonged.
- It can lead to a decrease in the volume of blood returning to the heart, which can result in serious cardiovascular complications.

Isotonic exercise, however, develops muscle throughout the full range of movement. This type of muscle contraction has no worrying side effects and will shape your body in the way you want. We will concentrate on isotonic exercise in this chapter.

RESISTANCE TRAINING FOR STRENGTH AND ENDURANCE

Principles of resistance training

Some muscles are exercised every time we stand or walk. Others need more specific exercises to get them working. A resistance training programme aims to work all the major muscle groups of the body in the most effective way.

A number of basic principles apply to all forms of resistance training. The principle of **overload** means that in order to gain in strength, one needs to stress the muscle or muscle group beyond the point to which it is normally stressed. A new manual job which seems

Building muscular strength and endurance

unbearably tiring at first becomes much more manageable within a few weeks. This is an everyday example of the body responding to overload.

The principle of **progressive resistance** means that the muscle will gradually adapt if resistance is progressively increased. Greek mythology tells the story of Milo of Crotona who wanted to be the strongest man in the world. When he was a young man he began lifting a newborn bull once a day, and continued this daily ritual until the bull had achieved full size. Milo became famous as the man who could lift a fully grown bull. But he did what anybody could do: took advantage of the principle of progressive resistance. As the weight of the bull increased so his muscles gradually adapted and grew in strength.

Modern resistance training programmes try to exploit these principles — overload and progressive resistance — to work and shape muscles in the most effective way.

Terms used in resistance training programmes

Before commencing a strength/endurance programme, we need to define some of the jargon used in resistance training: reps, sets, circuits, spotters.

- A repetition or **rep** is one complete execution of an exercise, from starting position, through the movement, back to starting position again.

- A **set** is the required number of repetitions. There will be few reps in a set if you are doing strength work, more if you are doing endurance work. You will generally do more than one set for either type of work.

- A **circuit** is a round of a number of different exercises. You might complete more than one circuit of exercises in one workout.

- A **spotter** is a partner to assist you when training for strength. Strength training requires you to lift the heaviest weights you can lift, so can be potentially dangerous. A spotter will hand the weight to you once you are in the correct starting position, will control the weight during the lift and take the weight at the end when the muscle is tired and an accident is most likely to occur. Without spotters, even the most experienced weight trainer can get into trouble.

MUSCULAR STRENGTH OR MUSCULAR ENDURANCE

The terms muscular strength and muscular endurance are often used interchangeably but this is incorrect since each has a distinct meaning. **Muscular strength** refers to the ability of the muscle or muscle group to exert force, whereas **muscular endurance** is the ability of the muscle or muscle group to sustain prolonged exercise.

- Muscular strength means how much force you can exert in all out, short-term effort.
- Muscular endurance means how many times you can work a particular muscle in a long-term activity at less than maximum effort.

Those training for strength use heavy weights and few repetitions. This is also the way body-builders train, as an increase in strength leads to an increase in muscle size. But those who do not wish to increase the size of their muscles should not be afraid to use weights. Improved muscular endurance will result in well-toned, shapely (rather than bulging) muscles. This is achieved by using light weights and performing lots of reps.

The terms 'light' or 'heavy' are obviously relative as what is heavy for one person is light for another. It is generally accepted that a strength-training programme will use not more than 8 repetitions of an exercise in each set, with the last rep requiring all out effort (hence the need for a spotter). Once 8 repetitions can be completed with relative ease, it is time to increase the resistance.

When training for muscular endurance, on the other hand, a minimum number of repetitions in a set would be 8 to 10. This could be increased to 20 repetitions, before increasing weight.

To summarise:

- Training for strength/increase in muscle size:
  Maximum number of repetitions   8
  Resistance   High
- Training for endurance/improved muscle tone:
  Maximum number of repetitions   20
  Resistance   Moderate

However, strength training should not be attempted until a reasonable level of muscular endurance has been attained.

MUSCLE SORENESS

There are two types of muscle soreness. One is felt immediately

Building muscular strength and endurance

following a bout of intense muscular exercise. This is transient although it may last for several hours, and it is usually minor. But the muscle soreness which is felt from 12 to 48 hours after the bout of exercise — called **delayed muscle soreness** — can be quite painful and considerable research has focussed on it. There is no need for this type of soreness.

People often express delight when they feel their muscles ache after a workout: 'If I feel it, it must be doing me good.' In fact, the opposite is the case. Soreness is usually a sign of having done too much, too soon, and it can interfere with your progress. A mild stiffness after exercise is to be expected if you have not trained for some time. Being unable to walk, however, is a cause for concern, not congratulation!

Delayed muscle soreness can be avoided by progressing your exercise programme carefully. Take it easy at the start and be slow to increase reps or weight. There is nothing to be gained by increasing too quickly. You are only fooling yourself, but you will find that you cannot fool your body.

Static stretching helps to prevent soreness and also provides relief to soreness when it is present.

STRENGTH/ENDURANCE EXERCISE PROGRAMME

The following exercises can all be done at home. Although the exercises are illustrated and explained using weights as resistance, ensure that you are able to perform them 'free' first of all. If it is some time since you exercised your muscles, you will probably find the resistance of gravity sufficiently taxing. Until you can do the 'free' exercise with perfect technique and complete ease, do not add weight.

When it comes to adding weight, you can improvise at first. A few bags of sugar or heavy books should provide the extra resistance you need. As you improve, you may want to invest in purpose-manufactured weights. Ankle weights, wrist weights, dumbells and barbells along with exercise benches can be purchased at any good sports shop.

It is possible to train for strength at home, but remember the principles of strength training. Unless you use few reps at maximum weight, any increases in strength or muscle size will be minimal. So you will need the help of a spotter. If you become serious about training for strength/body building, it will probably pay you to join a gymnasium (see below).

Squats

Muscle(s) worked: Quadriceps; hamstrings; gluteals (upper leg muscles and buttocks).

Starting position: Stand tall with feet slightly wider than hip width apart. Place your hands on your shoulders, elbows out to side.

Movement: Keeping your back flat throughout, head in line with spine, eyes forward while you slowly bend your knees controlling the movement down. Make sure the knees follow the same line as the toes and don't fall inwards. Return smoothly to the starting position, straightening (without locking) your knees.

Progression: Use a barbell, held across the shoulders/upper back with a wide grip. Increase reps.

Breathing: Breathe in as you go down, out as you come up.

Fig 15: Squats

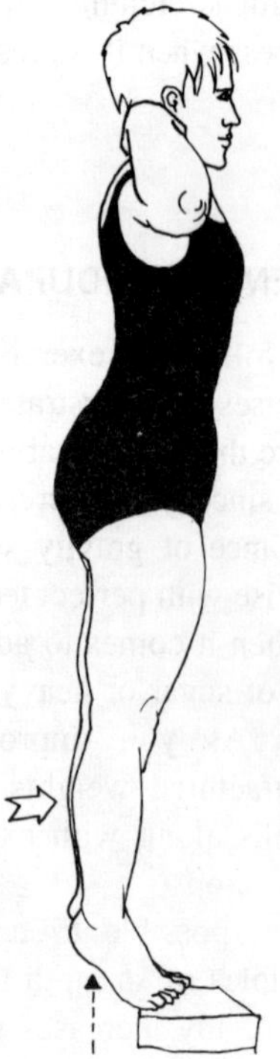

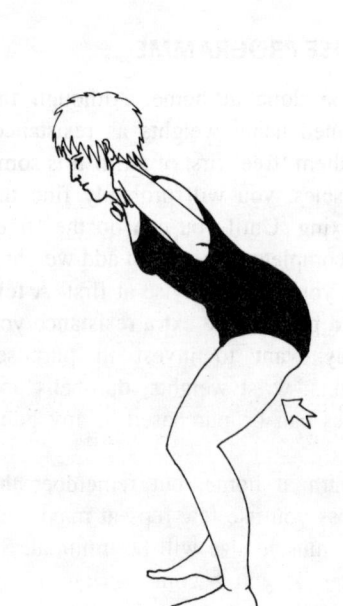

Fig 17: Heel raise

Building muscular strength and endurance

Leg raises

Muscle(s) worked: Gluteals; hamstrings; erector spinae (buttocks; back of thighs; lower back).

Starting position: Lie face down with head resting on hands.

Movement: Keeping hips to the floor lift right leg. Hold momentarily, then return to start under control. Repeat set with left leg.

Progression: Add weight. Increase reps.

Breathing: Breathe easily and regularly.

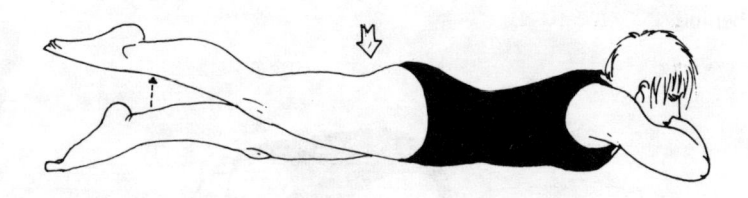

Fig 16: Leg raises

Heel raise

Muscle(s) worked: Gastrocnemius; soleus (calf muscles).

Starting position: As for squat, but with the balls of your feet resting on a block of wood (or telephone directory) heels on the floor.

Movement: Keeping legs straight, rise up on your toes, hold, then return to starting position.

Progression: Use barbell held across shoulders/upper back with a wide grip. Increase reps.

Breathing: Easy, regular breathing throughout.

Kneeling kick back

Muscle(s) worked: Hamstrings; gluteals (back of thigh and buttocks).

Starting position: On hands and knees, knees beneath hips, hands beneath shoulders.

Movement: Rounding back, bring right knee forward and head down so that knee and head almost touch. Push right leg back with a smooth action so that leg straightens parallel with floor. Ensure that hips remain facing floor and back does not arch. Repeat set on left leg.

Progression: Add ankle weight. Increase reps.

Breathing: Breathe out as you bring leg in, and in as you push leg behind.

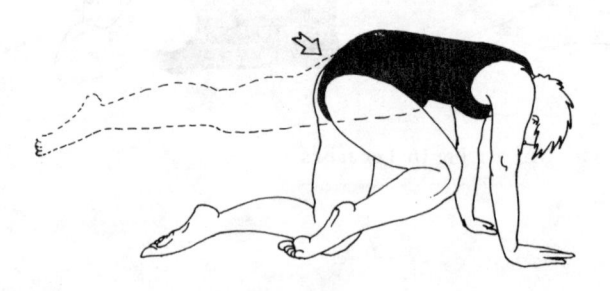

Fig 18: Kneeling kick back

Side leg lifts

Muscle(s) worked: Hip abductors (outer hip and thigh).

Starting position: Lie on right side with body held in a straight line from ankle through hip to shoulder. Rest head on right arm underneath. Hold left hand in front of chest, lightly supporting body weight.

Movement: Keeping hips facing forward, raise left leg so that knee and foot face forward. Avoid any tendency to roll forward or, more likely, backwards. Only lift as far as possible with hips facing forward. Hold foot at top of movement, then slowly lower to starting position. Repeat set on right side.

Building muscular strength and endurance 55

Progression: Add ankle weight. Increase reps.

Breathing: Breathe easily and regularly throughout.

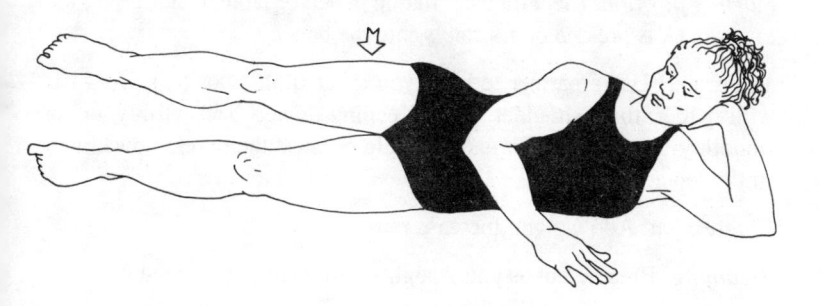

Fig 19: Side leg lifts

Lower leg lifts

Muscle(s) worked: Hip abductors (inner thigh).

Starting position: As for side leg lifts but bring left leg over and forward of lower leg.

Movement: Lift right leg from floor keeping right knee and right foot facing forward. Hold at top of movement then slowly lower. Repeat set on left side.

Progression: Add ankle weight. Increase reps.

Breathing: Breathe easily and regularly throughout.

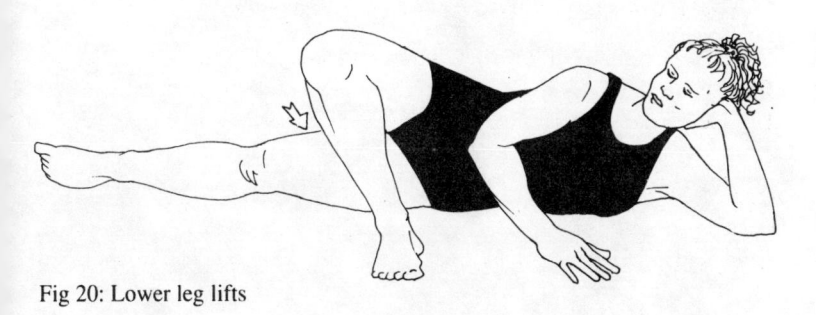

Fig 20: Lower leg lifts

Bench press: chest press on bench

Muscle(s) worked: Pectorals; Triceps; Anterior deltoid (muscles of the chest, back of upper arm, front of shoulder).

Starting position: Lie with back flat on bench or table, making sure the lower back is pressed comfortably into the bench.

Movement: Use a partner to hand you a bar in this position. Hold bar with wider than shoulder grip. Keeping lower back firmly down smoothly lower the bar to touch middle of chest then press upwards to straighten arms.

Progression: Add weight. Increase reps.

Breathing: Breathe out as you straighten arms, in as you bend.

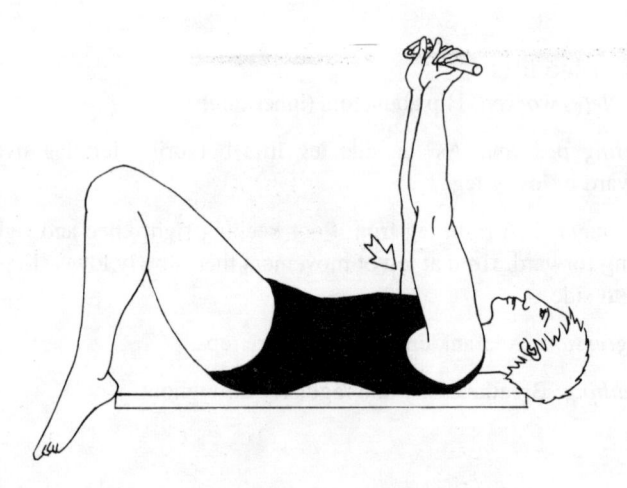

Fig 21: Chest press on bench

Building muscular strength and endurance

Bench flyes

Muscle(s) worked: Pectorals; anterior deltoid (chest and front of shoulder muscles).

Starting position: Lie on bench or table as in bench press but with wrists together above chest, hands lightly clenched, elbows bent slightly.

Movement: Keeping elbows slightly bent, bring arms out to side opening out chest as wide as possible. Smoothly return to starting position.

Progression: Add weights by holding dumbells. Increase reps.

Breathing: Breathe in as you lower arms, out as you raise them.

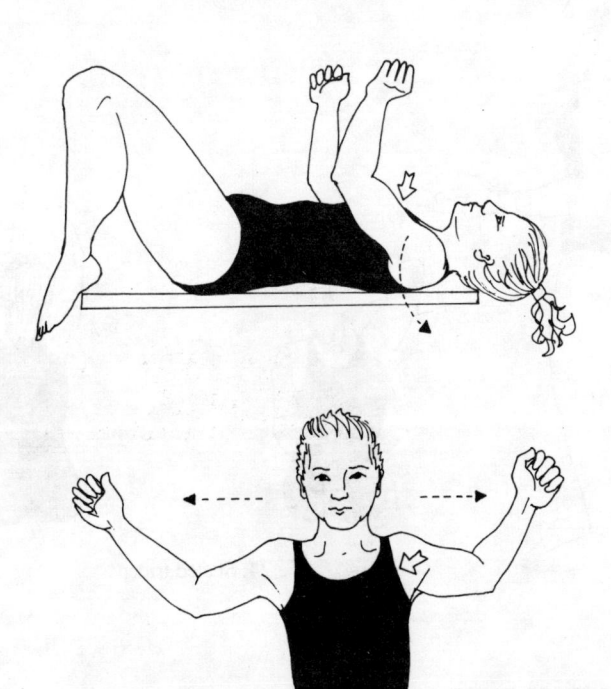

Fig 22: Bench flyes

Arm curl

Muscle(s) worked: Biceps (front of upper arm).

Starting position: Stand tall, feet shoulder width apart with knees slightly bent. Grip a bar with palms facing forward, hands slightly wider than hip width apart.

Movement: With upper arms close to the sides bend arms at elbow, smoothly lifting the bar to meet chest. The movement takes place solely in the elbow joint, not in the lower back or any other part of the body. Return to starting position under control.

Progression: Add weights to bar. Increase reps.

Breathing: Breathe in as you raise the bar and out as you lower it.

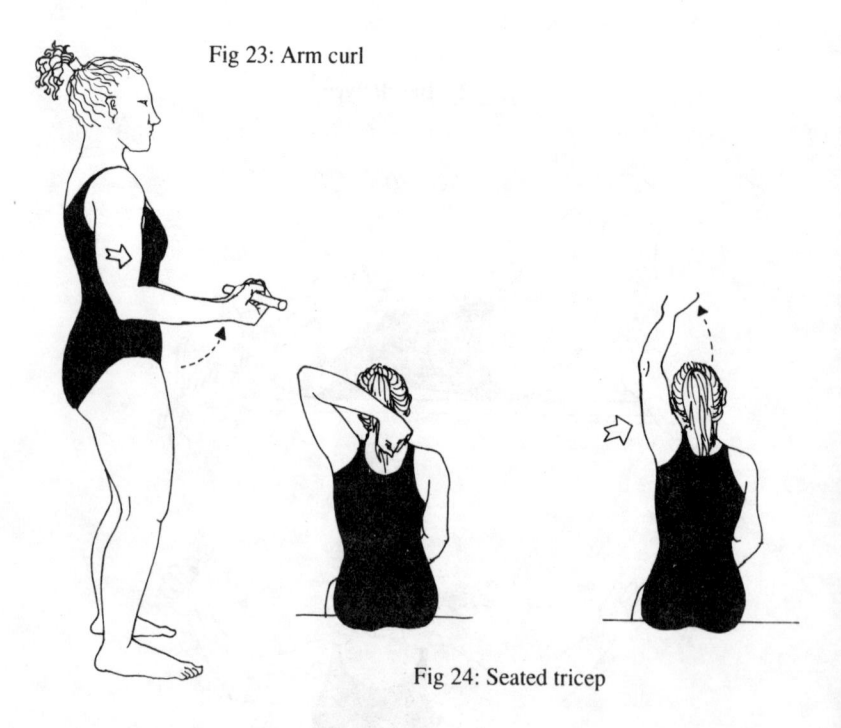

Fig 23: Arm curl

Fig 24: Seated tricep

Seated tricep press

Muscle(s) worked: Triceps (back of upper arm).

Starting position: Sit upright on bench or hard chair. Feet should be apart and flat on the floor to give firm base. Bring right arm straight overhead, then behind head so that right hand is almost touching the back of the neck.

Movement: Smoothly straighten arm at the elbow without moving upper arm. Again, movement takes place solely in the elbow joint. Return to starting position.

Progression: Add weight by holding dumbell. Increase reps.

Breathing: Breathe in as you straighten arm, out as you lower.

Seated shoulder press behind neck

Muscle(s) worked: Deltoids; trapezius; triceps (muscles of the shoulders, upper back, backs of upper arms).

Starting position: Sit on bench or hard chair with bar resting lightly across shoulders/upper back and held with a wide grip.

Movement: Smoothly press the barbell upward, straightening arms. Return under control.

Progression: Add weight to bar. Increase reps.

Breathing: Breathe in as you straighten, out as you lower.

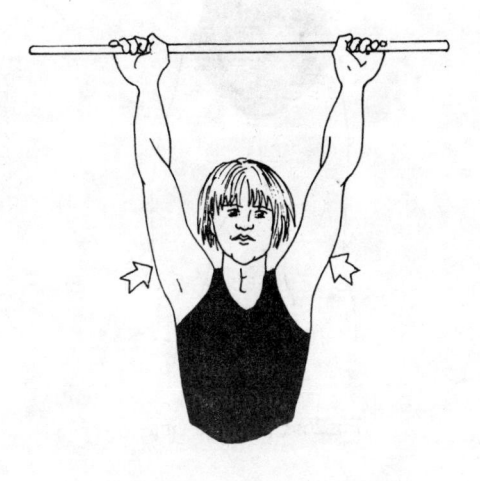

Fig 25: Seated shoulder press behind neck

Upright rowing

Muscle(s) worked: Deltoids; trapezius; biceps (muscles of the shoulders, upper back and front of upper arm).

Starting position: Stand tall holding bar with wrists facing body, arms and shoulders relaxed. Hands should be approximately two thumbs' distance apart.

Movement: From this position pull the bar upward to neck height leading with the elbows. Lower to starting position under control.

Progression: Add weight to bar. Increase reps.

Breathing: Breathe in as you raise the bar, out as you lower.

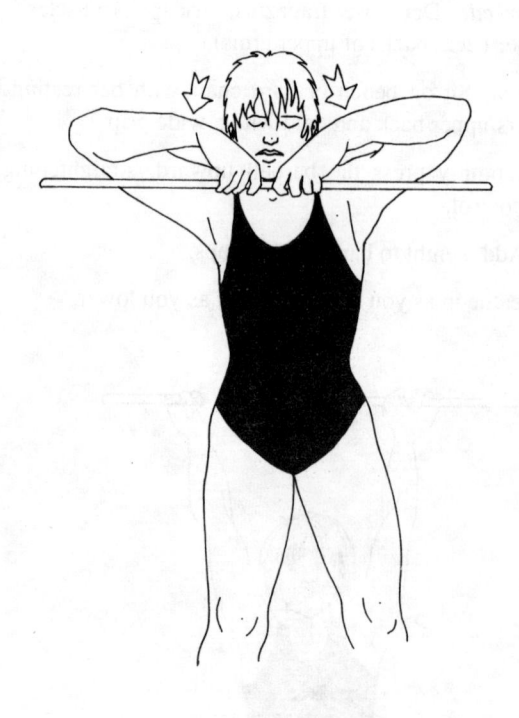

Fig 26: Upright rowing

Building muscular strength and endurance

Lateral raises

Muscle(s) worked: Deltoids; trapezius (muscles of shoulders and upper back).

Starting position: Stand tall with feet hip width apart, fists lightly clenched and held by sides, wrists facing inwards and elbows slightly bent.

Movement: Raise both arms out to the sides and up just above shoulder height. Keep elbows slightly bent throughout. Lower under control. The movement takes place solely in the shoulder joint. Resist any inclination to lean forwards or backwards.

Progression: Add weight by holding dumbells in hands. Increase reps.

Breathing: Breathe in as you raise arms, out as you lower them.

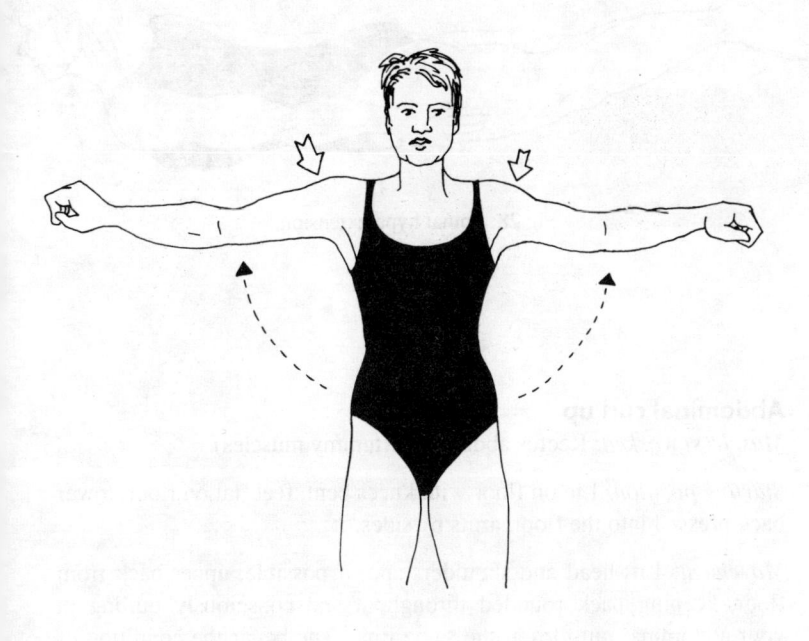

Fig 27: Lateral raises

Spinal hyperextension

Muscle(s) worked: Erector spinae; gluteals; hamstrings (muscles of the back, the buttocks and the backs of the thighs).

Starting position: Lie face down on a mat with hands resting on the small of your back.

Movement: Keeping spine long, raise chest from floor. Hold uppermost position momentarily. Return to starting position under control.

Progression: Rest hands behind head, elbows out to side. Increase reps.

Breathing: Breathe out as you lift, in as you lower.

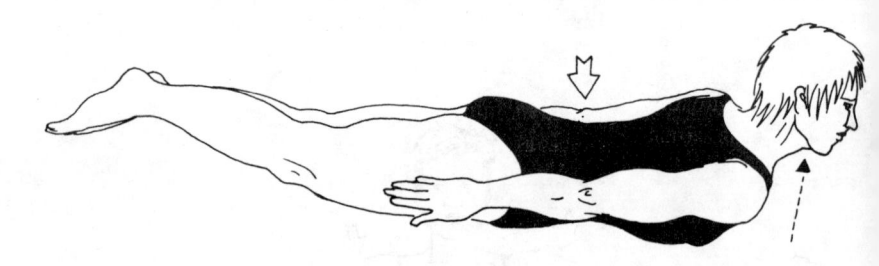

Fig 28: Spinal hyperextension

Abdominal curl up

Muscle(s) worked: Rectus abdominus (tummy muscles).

Starting position: Lie on floor with knees bent, feet flat on floor, lower back pressed into the floor, arms by sides.

Movement: Lift head and shoulders and, if possible, upper back from floor, keeping back rounded throughout and consciously pulling in your abdominal muscles at the same time. The better the condition of these muscles the more of your back you will be able to lift, but there is little advantage in going beyond the position illustrated. Hold final position momentarily. Lower under control still keeping a rounded back.

Progression: Rest arms behind head, elbows out to side. Increase reps.

Building muscular strength and endurance 63

Breathing: Breathe out as you lift and contract the abdominals, in as you lower and release the contraction.

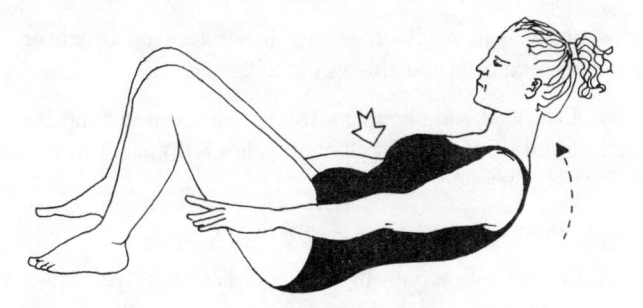

Fig 29: Abdominal curl-up

Reverse abdominal curl

Muscle(s) worked: Rectus abdominus (tummy muscles).

Starting position: Lie on back, hands behind head and elbows out to side, ankles crossed.

Movement: Pull in the abdominal muscles so that the knees are brought back towards the chest. This is a small movement, and it is easy to allow momentum or other muscles to do the work of the abdominals. Concentrate on pulling in tight.

Progression: Instead of pulling knees towards chest, use the abdominals to push upwards towards ceiling. Again the movement is small and most of the back remains on the floor.

Breathing: Breathe out as abdominals are contracted, in as they are released.

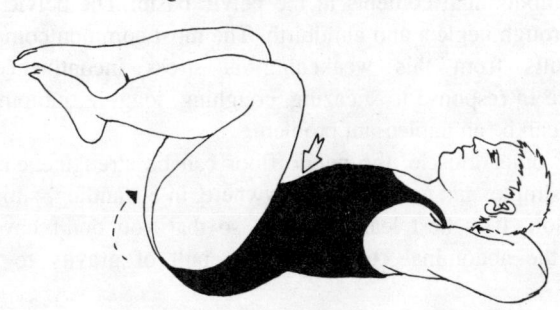

Fig 30: Reverse abdominal curl-up

Diagonal crunch

Muscle(s) worked: Rectus abdominus; obliques (tummy and waist muscles).

Starting position: Lie on floor, resting lower legs on bench or low chair, hands behind head and elbows out to the side.

Movement: Lift head and shoulders from floor as in curl up but this time twist as you lift until right elbow touches left knee. Lower under control. Repeat other side.

Progression: Increase reps.

Breathing: Breathe out as you lift and contract, in as you lower and release.

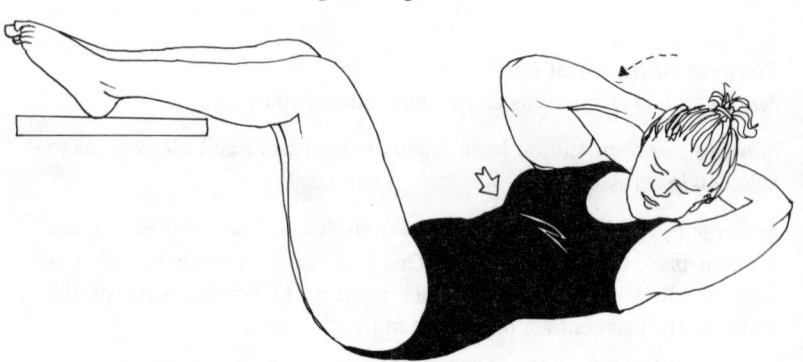

Fig 31: Diagonal crunch

For women only — pelvic floor lifts

Pelvic lifts exercise muscles which tend to cause most women problems at some stage of their lives. These muscles are the perineum muscles or the **pelvic floor** and are responsible for holding the lower part of the abdominal contents in the pelvic basin. The pelvic floor weakens through neglect and childbirth. The most common complaint which results from this weakening is stress incontinence — incontinence in response to sneezing, coughing, jogging, jumping etc — and this can be an unpleasant problem.

Like any other muscle, the pelvic floor can be strengthened. The exercise is simple, and can be done anywhere, in a standing, sitting or lying position. It is best learned lying, so that you don't have the weight of the abdominal contents or the pull of gravity to work against.

Building muscular strength and endurance

Lie on your back with your knees bent and feet flat on the floor, feet hip distance apart. Draw up the pelvic floor and grip with the sphincter muscles of the anus, urethra and vagina until you feel the inside passages tighten up. Hold for two to three seconds, then release.

You can test whether you are doing the exercise correctly by trying to stop your urine flow when on the toilet. Once you are happy that your technique is correct, you can incorporate this exercise into your daily life as much as possible.

CHOOSING A GYMNASIUM

Some people find it difficult to motivate themselves to exercise alone at home. Others don't have the space to set up a pleasant training environment in their house. And others become very interested in weight training and want to include a wider range of equipment into their routine. For such people, joining a gymnasium or fitness centre is usually a good idea.

It is possible to tell a good gym from a bad one in minutes, if you know what to look for. Don't be conned by appearances. That plush, well-decorated establishment may cut corners on staffing budgets and not provide qualified instruction. Fitness centres should be judged by three criteria: environment, equipment and facilities, and instruction.

Environment

A good workout environment is clean, spacious and airy, not small and poky. One of the main aspects of a gym environment is that there should be sufficient space to work out without feeling uncomfortably (or dangerously) close to somebody else. Good ventilation is another essential.

Equipment and facilities

Some of the facilities on offer may for example include sauna, jacuzzi, steam rooms, and sunbeds. While these can contribute to your enjoyment, more important is the type of exercise machinery available in the gym.

The most dramatic advance in the exercise equipment world was the variable resistance revolution pioneered by Nautilus. These machines adapt to muscle movement in a way which makes them far more effective than old-fashioned, pulley-style machines. So before joining a gym ask if the equipment uses a variable resistance system.

Instruction
The following are some instructional points to look for:
1. Before commencing a programme, each person should receive **medical screening**.
2. A **fitness assessment** should then given, analysing aerobic fitness, strength and muscular endurance and flexibility as well as weight, measurements and body fat.
3. **Individual attention** should be given at all times, not just on a first visit. An instructor should be able to keep an eye on members, and should constantly correct their posture, technique etc in a tactful way.
4. Programmes should provide for **re-assessment** and be regularly upgraded as improvements are made.
5. The instructor should know the basics of anatomy and exercise physiology, and apply them. Don't be afraid to check **qualifications**.

5
Improving Your Flexibility

In Chapter 4 we saw how the body moves by the action of the muscles. Muscles contract and lengthen, causing the bones to which they are attached to move.

Muscles work in pairs to achieve this miracle of movement. When the working muscle (**agonist**) shortens, its opposing muscle (**antagonist**) lengthens. For example, when you bend your elbow, the bicep muscle (the agonist) at the front of your upper arm shortens, while the triceps (the antagonist) at the back lengthens. As you straighten the opposite happens.

THE IMPORTANCE OF STRETCHING

Muscles are continually contracting in order to effect movement. This can cause tension to build up in the muscle, particularly those which are used regularly, like the leg muscles in walking. Stretching is the means by which these muscles are lengthened, easing tension and returning their flexibility.

To contract and shorten is a muscle's major function. A muscle needs strength to achieve this as we saw in Chapter 4. But length is equally important. If an antagonist muscle is short, and incapable of lengthening as the agonist contracts, muscle damage can occur.

If a muscle is continually contracted, without being lengthened by stretching, friction may be caused in the antagonist, resulting in either **muscle tears** or chronic injury such as **tendinitis**. The connection of the muscle onto the bone can also be irritated by this shortening of muscle causing problems like shin splints.

Chapter 2 illustrated how stretching will prepare your muscles for strenuous movement in the warm-up phase of a workout, and help reduce muscle soreness by relaxing your muscles afterwards in the cool-down.

A regular stretching programme, which includes all the major muscle groups, will make your whole body more flexible and mobile. Short, stiff muscles are one of the major contributors to poor posture, so stretching can improve this important area too.

A further reason for stretching is that natural muscle shrinkage with age tends to result in problems of stiffness and lack of mobility. A regular stretching programme can help to alleviate these problems.

However, stretching will *not* develop aerobic fitness, improve the strength/endurance of muscles, or burn fat. So stretching exercises must be combined with an aerobic and strength/endurance programme for all-round fitness.

Summary of reasons for stretching
- To decrease risk of muscle injury
- To increase mobility and allow for freer and easier movement.
- To improve relaxation and decrease stress by reducing muscle tension.
- To make strenuous movements easier by preparing the muscles for activity (warm-up).
- To prevent muscle soreness by restoring length to the muscle after contraction during exercise (cool-down).
- To improve posture.
- To decrease pain and mobility problems associated with ailments such as arthritis and chronic muscle tension.
- To improve blood circulation by allowing free flow of blood through relaxed muscles of the body.
- To develop body awareness.

Dangers of ballistic stretching
Ballistic or 'bounce' stretching deserves a mention here because it has been popularised, notably through Jane Fonda's original exercise workouts; it is still often recommended by unqualified exercise teachers and coaches.

Bounce or ballistic stretching is where the muscle is taken to the end of its range of motion and then pushed beyond that in a bouncing rhythm. Its proponents claim that it improves flexibility, but it is both ineffective and dangerous.

It is not difficult to see how bouncing can cause damage to overstretched muscle. And the risk is certainly not worth taking because certain physiological reactions ensure that bouncing does not improve flexibility. To understand this, it is necessary to examine a process called the **stretch reflex**.

All the muscle fibres contain nerve endings (**muscle spindles**) whose main function is to send messages back from the muscle, giving information about its state of stretch. If the muscle fibres are stretched too far (by bouncing or overstretching) the muscle spindle activates the stretch reflex — a protective reflex which causes the muscle to contract. It is an involuntary action, similar to the way your body reacts when you accidentally touch something hot.

So bouncing or overstretching causes a contraction of the muscle, tightening and shortening the very muscles you want to lengthen. The faster or more forceful the stretch, the faster and more forceful the reflex contraction of the stretched muscle.

The stretch reflex is only part of the muscle's response to stretching. Once a muscle is stretched to its full extent and held there for 6 seconds or more, a second reflex action called the **inverse stretch reflex** is brought into play. This reflex causes the antagonist muscle to that being stretched to relax, allowing the muscle to be further stretched without damage.

Ballistic actions are bounced, not held, so they are not extended for long enough to gain the benefits of the inverse stretch reflex. Ballistic stretching is, therefore, not just dangerous, but ineffective too.

Static stretching

Effective stretching, on the other hand, uses a technique called static stretching — the gradual stretching of a muscle to a position where it is held without bouncing for 10 to 30 seconds. The muscle should not be taken beyond a point of mild discomfort.

Static stretching is a safe and effective way of stretching muscles and connective tissue. It involves no sudden movements, so the stretch reflex is not brought into play as with ballistic movements. It also has a beneficial effect on the inverse stretch reflex.

When you begin a stretch, spend 10 to 30 seconds in the easy stretch. Go to the point of mild tension — and hold. Relax as you hold the stretch and the tension should subside. If not, ease it slightly and find a degree of tension that is comfortable.

When you feel the tension subside, move a fraction of an inch further until, once again, you feel mild tension in the muscle. Again, hold for 10 to 30 seconds. At first, you will need to count the seconds, but as you become accustomed to stretching, you will be able to stretch by the way the muscle feels.

Breathing should be controlled and rhythmical during a stretch. Don't hold your breath.

Checklist of rules for stretching

1. Warm up before stretching.
2. Breathe slowly, deeply and evenly.
3. Do not stretch to the point where breathing becomes unnatural.
4. Do not overstretch, particularly in early stages.
5. Hold the stretch in a comfortable position
6. Concentrate on the area being stretched, relaxing all other muscles.
7. Feel tension subside as the stretch is held.
8. Once the muscle relaxes, move a little further into the stretch returning to the point of mild tension. Hold.
9. Stretch regularly (3 times per week at least to improve overall flexibility).

STRETCHING PROGRAMME

When performing each of the following stretches, use the static stretch technique:

- Find the position of mild tension, and hold for 10 to 30 seconds until you feel the tension subside.
- Once the tension eases, move the stretch a fraction of an inch further, and hold for a further 10 to 30 seconds.
- Relax all other muscles in the body, concentrating on the muscle that is being stretched.

Improving your flexibility

Gastrocnemius (upper calf) stretch

Starting position: Stand, leaning against a wall at arm's length, right leg forward with knee bent, left leg behind with the foot facing directly forward towards the wall. Your body weight is resting on the right leg.

Movement: Keeping the upper body relaxed, gently ease the hips forward towards the wall, until you feel a stretch in the calf muscle. Repeat with other leg.

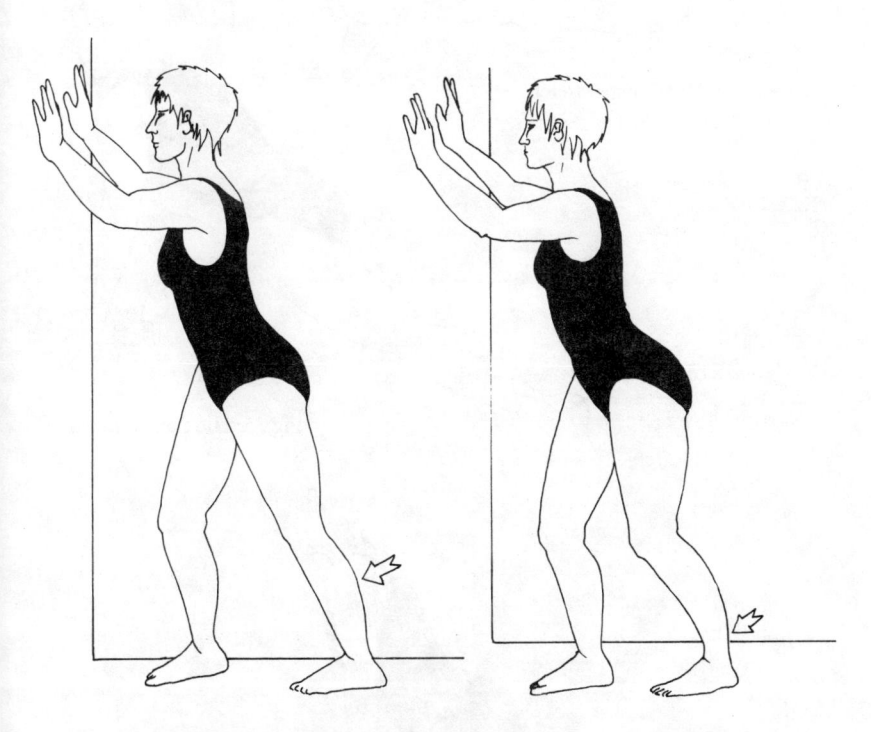

Fig 32: Gastrocnemius stretch

Fig 33: Soleus stretch

Soleus (lower calf) stretch

Starting position: As above, but with left leg bent.

Movement: With knee bent, ease hips forward. You should feel the stretch move down into the lower part of the calf muscle. Repeat other leg.

Fig 34: Quadriceps stretch

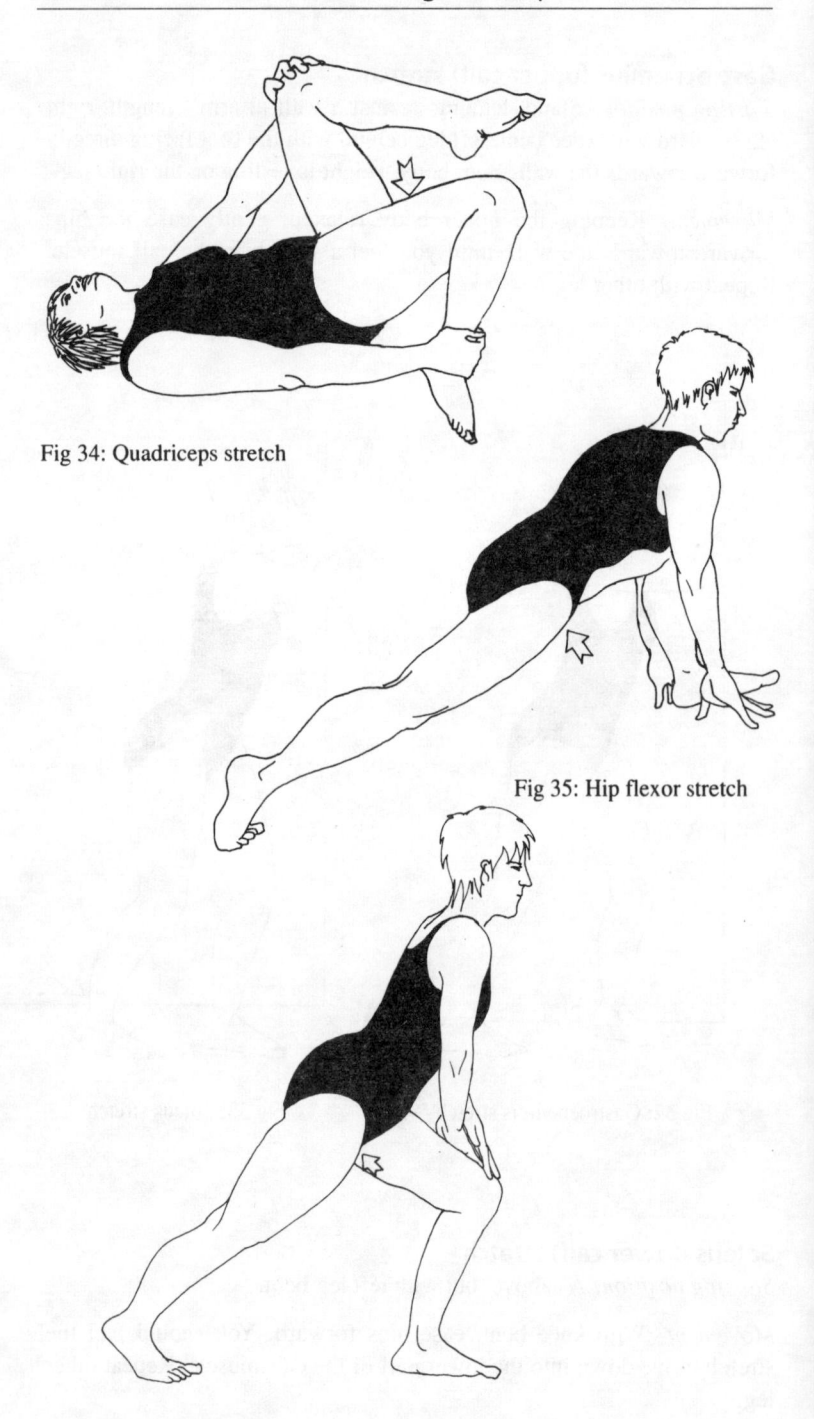

Fig 35: Hip flexor stretch

Improving your flexibility

Quadriceps (front of thigh) stretch
Starting position: Lie on the floor, on your side, right knee bent towards the chest held by right hand (to keep back rounded), left knee bent back, left hand holding left ankle. (Note: if your neck muscles are tense, you may find a cushion under your head makes this position more comfortable.)

Movement: Keeping left knee low, gently ease the left knee back until you feel a stretch at the front of your left thigh. Do *not* pull heel towards buttocks. Repeat other leg.

Hip flexor (front of hip) stretch
Starting position: Stand, feet together.

Movement: Take right leg behind, keeping hips forward, and bending left leg, until you feel a stretch in muscles at the top of the right leg. Your weight should rest on your left leg, with left knee directly over left heel. Repeat other leg.

Hamstring (back of thigh) stretch
Starting position: Lie on your back, right knee bent, foot flat on floor, left leg in air, supported by hands.

Movement: Gently ease the left leg back until you feel a stretch in the back of the thigh. The stretch is intensified by attempting to straighten the leg. Repeat other leg.

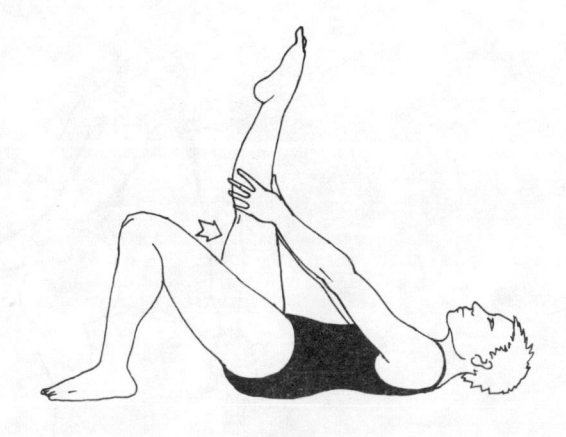

Fig 36: Hamstring stretch

Gluteal (buttocks) stretch

Starting position: As previous exercise, but with left knee bent so that left ankle rests on right thigh.

Movement: Gently lift right leg from floor until stretch is felt in left buttock. Repeat other leg.

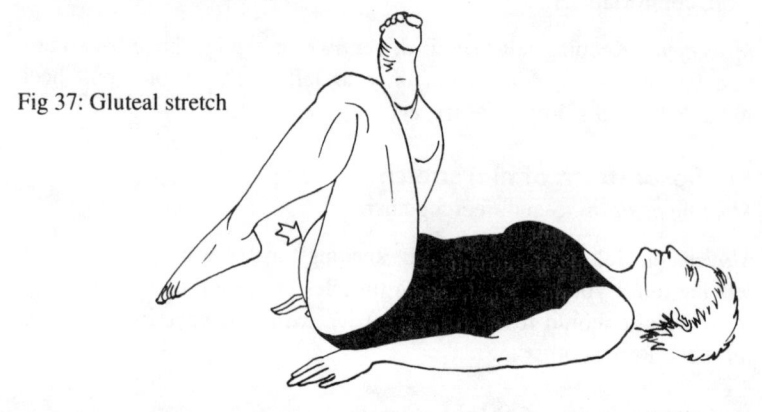

Fig 37: Gluteal stretch

Abductor (outer thigh) stretch

Starting position: Lie on your back, right knee bent into your chest, left knee bent so that the foot is flat on the floor.

Movement: Holding the right leg with your hand, draw the leg across towards the opposite shoulder, until you feel a stretch in the outer thigh of the right leg. Repeat other leg.

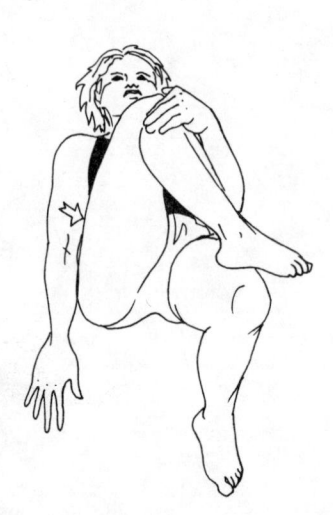

Fig 38: Abductor stretch

Improving your flexibility

Adductor (inner thigh) stretch

Starting position: Lie on your back, feet straight up in the air, hands supporting legs.

Movement: Gently open legs wide until you feel a stretch in the inner thighs. Use your hands to support the legs so that the muscle can lengthen without strain.

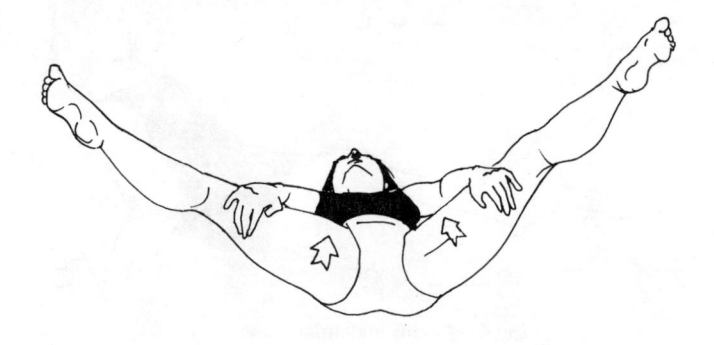

Fig 39: Adductor stretch

Erector spinae (lower back)

Starting position: Lie on back, knees bent into chest.

Movement: Using hands and holding under the knees, gently ease knees towards the chest, rounding the lower back.

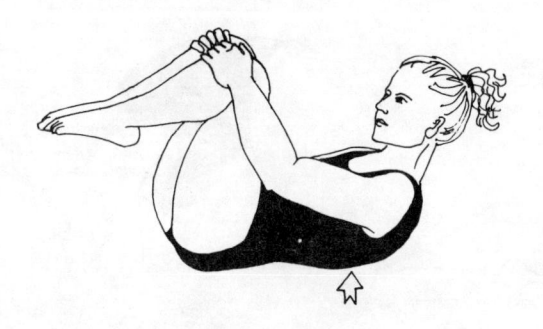

Fig 40: Erector spinae (lower back) stretch

Rectus abdominus (tummy muscles) stretch

Starting position: Lie on your front, arms bent with hands beneath your shoulders, head resting on floor.

Movement: Keeping head, neck and spine aligned, lift chest from floor until you feel a stretch in the abdominal muscles and rib cage. Use hands for support.

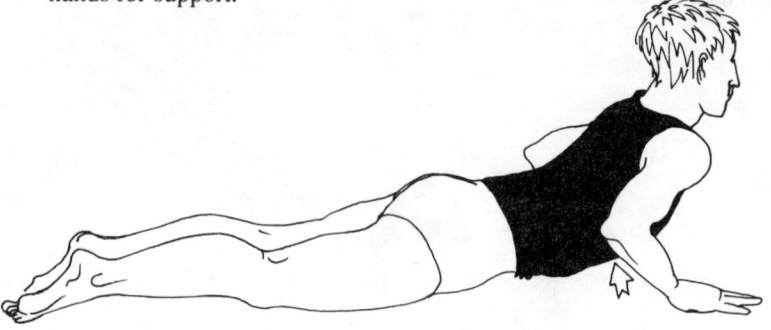

Fig 41: Rectus abdominus stretch

Erector spinae (upper back) stretch

Starting position: On hands and knees, back flat, shoulders over hands, hips over knees.

Movement: Pull tummy in and round back upwards like a cat, stretching the muscles of the upper back.

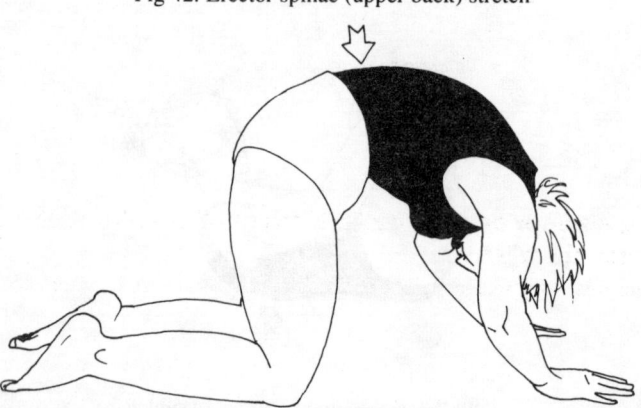

Fig 42: Erector spinae (upper back) stretch

Improving your flexibility

Posterior deltoid, trapezius (rear shoulder and upper back) stretch

Starting position: With shoulders relaxed and down, bend right arm across the upper body, so that right hand reaches behind left shoulder.

Movement: Use left hand to pull right elbow gently across, until you feel stretch over the upper back. Repeat other arm.

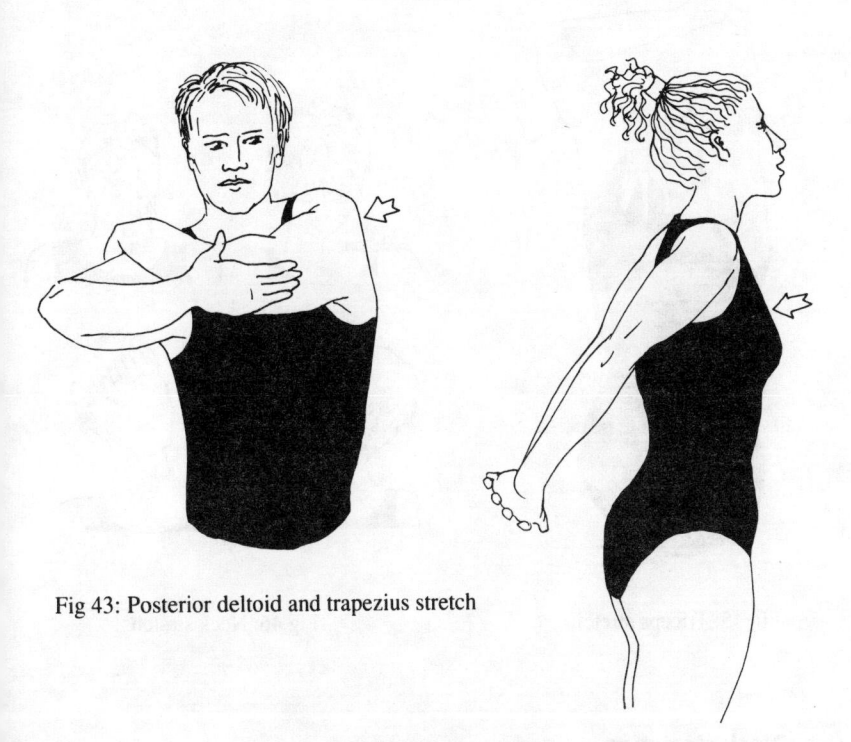

Fig 43: Posterior deltoid and trapezius stretch

Fig 44: Biceps, anterior deltoid and pectoral strecth

Biceps, anterior deltoid, pectoral (front of arm, front of shoulder, chest) stretch

Starting position: Clasp hands behind your back, keeping your elbows straight.

Movement: Lift arms back behind you, bringing shoulderblades together, until you feel a stretch over the front of your shoulder.

Triceps (back of arm) stretch

Starting position: Lift right arm over head, and bend elbow so that your right hand is behind your head.

Movement: With left hand, pull the elbow towards your head, until you feel the stretch at the back of the right arm. Repeat other arm.

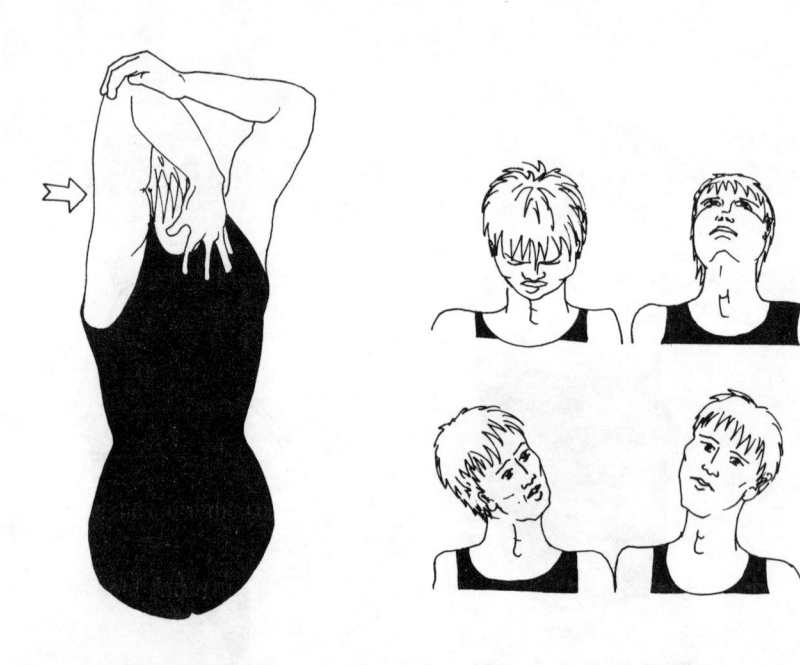

Fig 45: Triceps stretch

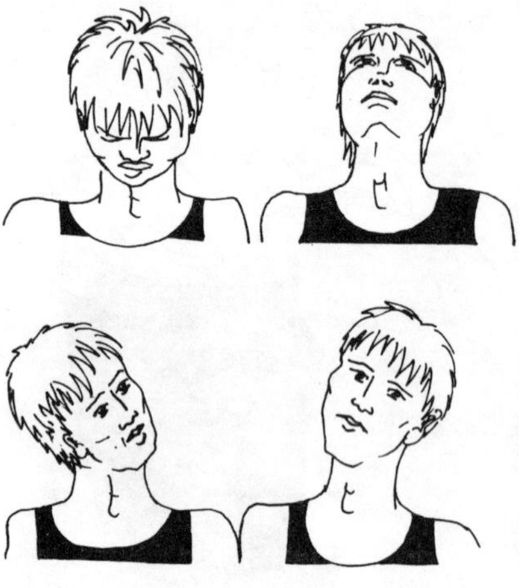

Fig 46: Neck stretch

Neck stretches

Starting position: Stand tall, chin centred, neck long.

Movement: Bend head forward, tilt head upwards, to the right side and to the left. Hold each position until you feel stretch in the neck muscles.

When doing a complete body workout — aerobic exercise strength/endurance work and flexibility — it is usually best to leave flexibility work to the end. At this stage, all the muscles will have worked vigorously and will therefore be warm and amenable to stretching.

Improving your flexibility

RELAXATION

A perfect end to a vigorous workout is a relaxation session. This will eliminate any residual muscle tension and leave you feeling mentally, as well as physically, refreshed. But, of course, relaxation techniques can be practised at any time. Once you are familiar with the method, you will find it easy to apply it in appropriate situations; for example, when under stress, or trying to sleep.

One easily learned technique of relaxation is aimed at recognising the feelings produced by tension. Lie on your back wearing loose, comfortable clothing. Make sure the room is comfortably warm. You can also darken the room and put on some slow music if you wish.

The technique is to tense a specific area of the body, hold for about 20 seconds, then relax; then tense a larger segment, hold for 20 seconds, relax and so on. Concentrate on feeling the tension during the hold period and then feeling the tension leave the area as you relax.

Begin by breathing deeply, in through the nose and out through the mouth. Draw each breath way down into the centre of the body and keep breathing deeply throughout. (Do not hold your breath during the tension period.)

Tighten and relax body parts in the following sequence:

Right toes
Left toes
Right foot
Left foot
Right leg below knee
Left leg below knee
Right leg below hip
Left leg below hip
Both legs together
Buttocks
Abdomen
Abdomen and buttocks together

Right fingers
Left fingers
Right arm below elbow
Left arm below elbow
Right arm below shoulder
Left arm below shoulder
Both arms together
Chest
Upper back and neck
Face
Entire body (twice)

Remain, breathing deeply and feeling all the muscles of the body relaxed and heavy, for as long as you wish.

6
Safety and Injury

Safety in exercise is a relatively recent preoccupation. Until recently, everybody assumed that exercise *per se* was a good thing. The nature of the exercise, or the nature of the exerciser was not questioned.

Exercise routines were rarely designed for the unfit audience at which they were aimed. They tended to be derived from the programmes of athletes, sportspeople or dancers. And exercise was promoted in the media by people (usually celebrities) with few or no qualifications in exercise anatomy and physiology.

It was possibly journalists' notorious resistance to an active lifestyle which started the general public, and exercise instructors, thinking about safety. When aerobic-related injuries started occurring in the early 1980s, and when Jim Fix, running guru, died in 1984, the press leaped to conclusions. EXERCISE IS DANGEROUS screamed the headlines. And exercise instructors and researchers had to re-think their approach.

The truth, of course, is not that exercise itself is dangerous, but that over-strenuous, inappropriate exercise can cause injury and even, in extreme cases, death.

So we must take safety seriously. In an ideal world, everybody would be fit and well, and able to do most exercises without harming themselves. But the average person does not fit this ideal. Years of poor posture, and poor exercise and eating habits take their toll and must be taken into account.

CONTRAINDICATED EXERCISE

There is no such thing as an inherently good or bad exercise. So much depends on what you are trying to achieve. What is acceptable for the professional dancer or weightlifter, for example, may not be right for you. The costs and benefits of an exercise must be considered before

Safety and injury

choosing it for our exercise routine.

To do this you need a basic knowledge of how the body moves and works, ie anatomy and physiology. This is why the anatomical and physiological theory behind the exercises in this book are explained in some detail. You may be impatient to get on with the exercises and find some of the theory difficult or boring, but it is important to understand it before you start. Only then can you know what you are doing with your body, and why.

A **contraindicated exercise** is one which is medically inadvisable for a particular individual. Some of the conditions discussed in Chapter 1, such as coronary heart disease for example, are contraindications to strenuous exercise under normal conditions. There are a few exercises which have been popular for years but which are now recognised as being contraindicated for most people — they work contra to the body's natural potential for movement. Because these exercises are so popular, being constantly regurgitated in newspapers, books and magazines, they are worth noting here.

The reason for concern and an alternative exercise are also noted.

Straight leg sit up

This exercise is most frequently recommended to 'strengthen the abdominals'. While the abdominals do work during this exercise, they are not being worked in the most effective way. This is because of the hip flexor muscles, which are attached to the lower lumbar vertebrae

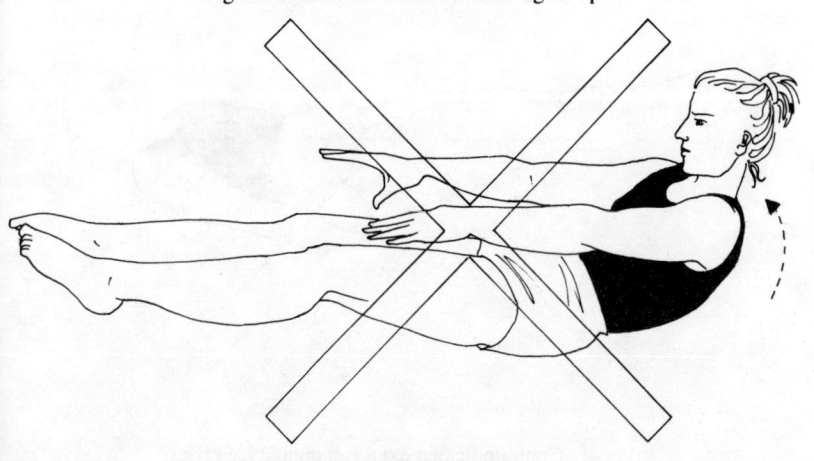

Fig 47: Contraindicated exercise: leg sit up

and to the head of each thigh bone. Their action is to flex the hip joint, an action which occurs every time you walk a step. Because of this, they are well exercised, strong muscles.

If the tummy muscles are weak, the hip flexors take over during a straight leg sit up. Because they are attached to the lumbar spine, the lower back arches and the tummy muscle bulge and stretch — the very *opposite* to what you hope to achieve.

- **Alternative: Bent knee curl-up** (fig 29, p.63).
  By bending the knees, the hip flexors are relaxed and the abdominals can work in isolation. Most of the abdominal work in a sit-up is in the first 30 degrees of the movement. There is no need to go beyond this point unless you are specifically interested in working the muscle through the full range of movement.

Double leg raises

Here, too, the hip flexors come into play. While the abdominals may work isometrically to hold the legs — you can often feel this happening — they are bulging and stretching as they hold. You may also feel pain in the lower back as the stronger hip flexor muscles pull on the lumbar vertebrae causing the back to arch from the floor.

- **Alternative: reverse curl-ups** (fig 30, p.63).
  Lie on back, hands behind head, head and shoulders relaxed on floor. Lift feet above hips, ankles crossed and knees facing out to

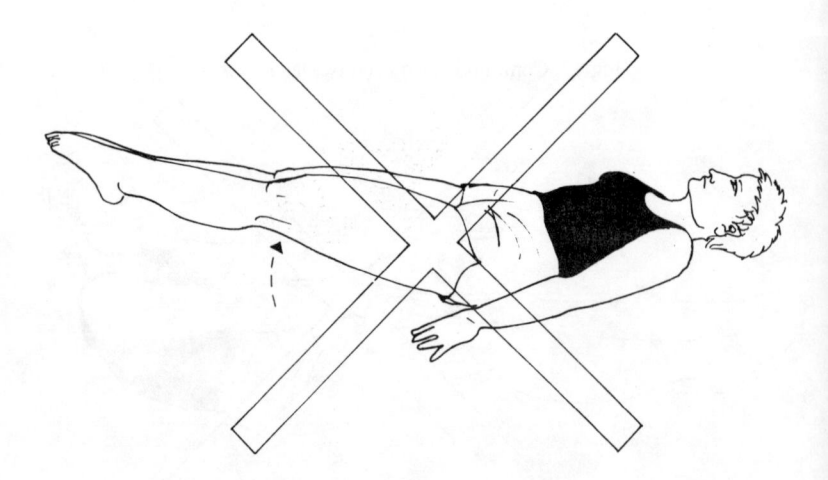

Fig 48: Contraindicated exercise: double leg raises

side. This is your starting position. Contract the tummy muscles and breathe out so that the knees move slightly towards the chest. Hold for two seconds and release. Note: It is not a 'rolling' movement; the contraction of the abdominals is what pulls the knees back.

Swinging toe touches

This is often done in a warm up. The legs are straight with the upper body in a bent forward position while the arms swing side to side to touch the opposite feet. The aim of the exercise is said to be to stretch the hamstrings and warm up the trunk area.

This is another exercise which can have an adverse effect on the lower back. In a forward flexed position, the discs (which provide protection) between the lumbar vertebrae are compressed. Rotating the vertebrae from side to side in this position puts pressure on the intervertebral discs and also strains the ligaments of the lower back.

Neither is it an effective way to stretch the hamstrings. In this position, the hamstrings are weight bearing, straining to hold the weight of the body in position. You are therefore trying to stretch a contracted muscle, not a good idea.

- **Alternative: to stretch the hamstring** (fig 36, p.73).
  Lie on the back grasping the extended leg at the knee and pulling it gently towards the chest. (Rotation of the trunk — trunk twists — can be performed in an upright position without any detrimental effect.)

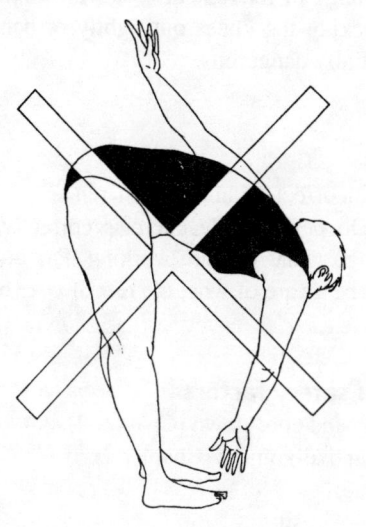

Fig 49: Contraindicated exercise: swinging toe touches

OTHER SAFETY ASPECTS

Exercise intensity

If an exercise is too intense, it will be at best tiring, at worst dangerous. But if it is not intense enough it is unlikely to do any good. Therefore you need to monitor the intensity at which you perform an exercise to ensure that the level of activity is appropriate to you, and to what you are trying to achieve. This is particularly important in relation to aerobic exercise.

Monitoring exercise intensity is largely a matter of 'listening' to your body. When working aerobically, checking heart rate is the best way of monitoring exercise intensity. Activity should take place at 60 to 85 per cent of maximum — see Chapter 3.

During strength/endurance work, pain is generally a reliable monitor. Any exercise which feels uncomfortable is inappropriate and repetitions or resistance should be reduced, or technique checked. Similarly, during flexibility work, stretches should be held to a point of mild tension only, never stretching beyond the point of pain.

Joints

As you work, consider the range of movement of the working joint. If it only flexes and extends, such as the knee joint, any movement which works it sideways could cause damage. Similarly, be careful at both ends of the range of movement — at full flexion or full extension of the knee. Locking the knees out tightly or bending then very deeply can be potentially dangerous.

Technique

Careless or incorrect technique can render an exercise dangerous or ineffective. Do perform the exercise correctly, concentrating on the muscle/body part that you are working. Pay attention to your starting position, and be aware of what the rest of your body is doing.

Checklist of safety factors

1. Warm-up and cool-down (Chapter 2).
2. Posture and alignment (Chapter 2).
3. Technique.
4. Exercise intensity
5. Contraindicated exercise.

Safety and injury

FACTORS AFFECTING INJURY

The importance of screening out individuals who are at risk of injury cannot be overstressed. The medical examination before you start should be orientated toward the intended sport or exercise activity; for example, the examination of a middle-aged jogger should be orientated toward the diagnosis of cardiovascular condition.

The following factors also affect susceptibility to injury and should be taken into account.

- **Fitness level**. Violent exercise for the unfit can be fatal. Remember that fitness is specific. A highly-trained weightlifter is not necessarily able to run a half marathon, and it may be dangerous for him to attempt to do so.
- **Body shape**. Excess body fat places strain on joints, muscles and circulatory system.
- **Age**. Susceptibility to cardiorespiratory problems, ligamental, muscular and tendon problems increases with age. Bones may become more brittle and arthritis more common. The very young can be vulnerable, too, as their bones, muscles and tendons are still developing and should not be placed under too much stress.
- **Environment** may also be a risk factor. Excess heat puts the cardiovascular system under stress. A cold environment increases vulnerability to muscle strains and tears. Playing fields, equipment and floor surfaces can all increase the likelihood of injury.

TYPES OF INJURY

At some stage most exercisers experience an exercise-related injury. Most injuries fall into two categories: exposed wounds or unexposed wounds.

Exposed wounds

- **Abrasions**: the skin is abraded or scraped against a rough surface. The outer layers of skin are torn away exposing numerous capillaries.
- **Lacerations**: a sharp or pointed object tears the tissue, giving the wound a deep, jagged-edged appearance.
- **Puncture wounds**: the skin and underlying tissues are punctured by a sharp, pointed object.
- **Incisions**: clean cuts which most frequently occur as the result of a direct blow over a sharp or poorly padded bone.

Unexposed wounds

- **Contusions**: bruises which are the result of traumatic blows to the body. Most are minor producing no more of a problem than localised soreness. Occasionally they can be major, involving deep tissue tears and haemorrhage.
- **Strains**: the muscle or adjacent tissue tears. A snapping sound may be heard, followed immediately by a sharp pain, with loss of function and severe weakness in the area. Frequently an indentation or cavity can be felt where the tissues have separated.
- **Sprains**: a stretching or tearing of the stabilising connective tissue of a joint, usually the result of a traumatic twisting. Blood and synovial fluid leak into the joint cavity, causing swelling and extreme tenderness, and limiting the range of motion.
- **Dislocations**: the joint is forced beyond its normal limitations, leading to immediate loss of limb function with swelling, tenderness and deformity of the joint.
- **Fractures**: broken bone. Fractures can be simple (a break in the bone without breaking through the skin) or compound (the bone extends through the outer layers of the skin.)

Other injuries

There are other injuries or problems which do not fall into these categories:

- **Muscle soreness**: delayed muscle soreness is generally the result of not graduating a programme, of doing too much, too soon.
- **Muscle cramps**: generally associated with a salt, potassium or calcium imbalance in a muscle.
- **Tendinitis**: usually the result of overuse; the tendon becomes inflamed.
- **Bursitis**: an inflammation of the bursa, generally caused by excessive shock impact.
- **Blisters**: generally the result of excessive friction between the skin and some external surface such as a shoe. The epidermis separates from the dermis and fluid accumulates between the two layers of skin.
- **Shin splints**: a sharp pain along the front of the shin bone. Shin splints can arise from lowered arches, separation of the muscle from the bone, hairline fractures of the bone, irritated membranes and other factors and is usually associated with overuse, or high-impact aerobic work on hard surfaces.

CARDIOVASCULAR COMPLICATIONS

Most of the information presented in this section is directed toward musculoskeletal injuries. But cardiovascular problems must also be considered.

The following warning signs may occur during or following strenuous exercise: Abnormal heart activity including irregular pulse, fluttering or palpitations in the chest or throat, sudden speeding or slowing of pulse, pain or pressure in the centre of the chest, arm or throat. Dizziness, lightheadedness, pallor, cold sweats or fainting. Regular nausea or vomiting after exercise.

Should you experience any of these symptoms during or following exercise, you should stop the activity and consult a doctor before resuming.

AVOIDING INJURY

Injuries fall into one of four categories: sudden traumatic, repeated traumatic, overuse or imbalance.

Sudden traumatic injury
Example: a severe muscle strain or bone fracture.

Prevention: minimise risk factors. All equipment used should be the right size and weight for you and in good condition. Training shoes should fit properly and be appropriate for the exercise activity — tennis shoes for tennis, jogging shoes for jogging, and so on. Playing surfaces should be checked over for possible danger before play. Heat and cold can cause injury unless taken into account. Time of day can also play a part; for example, running in the midday sun should be avoided as should the dangers of city jogging during rush hour traffic.

Repeated traumatic injuries
Example: a knee which is wrenched in one play in a football game and continuously subjected to trauma on subsequent plays until the player finally has to remove himself from the game.

Prevention: be familiar with the major types of injuries associated with your intended sports activity so that you can take steps to minimise the chances of injury occurring. For example, ankle sprains are one of the most common injuries in basket ball. As a result many basket ball players tape their ankles to increase stability in the ankle joint area.

Overuse injuries

These are injuries which result from repetitive movements where the individual isn't properly trained for that level of stress.

Prevention: allow your body to adapt to repetitive stress. Increasing training must be a gradual process, building up in easy stages, allowing recovery days and rest days. Exercise intensity should be closely monitored.

Imbalance injuries

Imbalance injuries are the result of postural imbalances, anatomical weaknesses and overdevelopment of certain muscle groups at the expense of others.

Prevention: awareness of posture and correct technique. Ensure that a strength/endurance programme is balanced, working opposing muscle groups equally.

FIRST AID

Any person involved in exercise activity of any type should have a working knowledge of first aid and be clear about the appropriate action to take in an emergency.

If the brain is deprived of oxygen it can survive normally for about four minutes before its cells die off, causing irreparable harm. When a person has been exercising hard, that time is considerably reduced — to as little as eighteen seconds! So you need to know how to act very swiftly to save an exerciser who has collapsed.

First aid is also vital for traumatic injuries to bones or muscles. With such injuries the length of time between onset of injury and initial treatment can frequently determine the required recovery time afterwards.

The only real way to learn first aid is to do a standard aid course, where you can practise the techniques on models until you perfect them. First aid saves lives and ideally should be taught in school. As this is not done, you owe it to yourself, and to your fellow exercisers, to familiarise yourself with the principles and techniques.

Find out who runs first aid courses locally: the British Red Cross Society, St John Ambulance and the Royal Life Saving Society all organise courses (see page 121 for addresses). Medical assistance should be obtained as soon as possible for any injury of a potentially serious nature.

Treatment of minor injury

For less serious injuries such as sprains, strains and exposed wounds of a minor nature, the RICE treatment is the usual procedure. RICE is an acronym for Rest, Ice, Compression and Elevation.

- **Rest**
  Once an injury has been sustained, all activity should cease immediately. Pain will be greatly reduced if the injured part is immobilised correctly.

- **Ice**
  Cold treatment is universally accepted as the simplest and safest immediate measure for relieving pain and reducing bruising and swelling in injured tissues. Ice can be applied by rubbing ice cubes over the inured area, dabbing the skin dry at intervals. A wet towel containing ice cubes can be wrapped round the injury. An injured hand or foot can be immersed in a bucket or bowl of iced water. Prolonged used of ice or direct contact between ice and skin can lead to an 'ice burn'. But there us no set time for ice application. If your skin is sensitive, you may only be able to tolerate a few minutes. Others can stand it for much longer. When the skin turns pink (white skins) or darkens in colour (dark skins) you have achieved the effects you want.

- **Compression**
  Supportive bandaging applied to the injury will reduce stress, prevent painful movement and help control swelling.

- **Elevation**
  Damaged tissue releases fluid. After an injury excess fluid can accumulate at the injury site unless measures are taken to promote its reabsorption into the normal blood flow systems. One measure is to position the injured part so that gravity can help the return flow of the fluid. For any swelling of the legs, you should try to rest as much as possible with your foot supported above the level of the hip. For swelling in the hand or lower part of the arm, a sling can hold the hand at shoulder level. If the swelling is in the upper arm it is necessary to lift the arm above the head at frequent intervals and flex the muscles. For swelling in the back or abdomen, you should lie flat as much as possible rather than remain standing.

Alternative activity

Many serious exercisers are reluctant to rest when suffering from a minor injury. But an injured area *must* have rest for a sufficient period of time so that healing can take place. Attempting to 'train through' an injury greatly prolongs the time needed for recovery.

If you must have some form of activity during convalescence, there are usually substitute movements which protect the injured area but allow appropriate activity. For example, if a distance runner sustains a knee or ankle injury, it would be foolish and medically unsound to continue with a running programme, but a good substitute activity could be pedalling a stationary bicycle, or swimming or jogging in water with the body submerged to the base of the neck.

Rehabilitation

Rehabilitation from a major injury should take place under the guidance of a medical professional, usually a sports' physiotherapist. A combination of strengthening exercises, mobility exercises and stretching will generally be recommended.

Other treatments include massage, heat treatment, taping, bracing and ultrasound, none of which should be self-administered. Taking your therapy into your own hands without appropriate advice and supervision will probably result in more harm than good.

The decision to return to training after a serious injury can only be made by a medical professional who is familiar with the injury and has been involved with the rehabilitation programme. Premature return to activity can result in a far more serious injury and a longer lay-off time.

In the case of less serious injury, don't return to exercise until the injured area is pain free. Movement should be normal without limps or hitches, and the full range of motion along with normal strength, power and endurance should be restored.

7
Mastering Your Diet and Nutrition

As millions die of starvation in the Third World, citizens of the 'developed' word grow fatter and fatter. Life insurance statistics show that we are clearly heavier than we were twenty years ago.

Excess weight is uncomfortable, unsightly and unhealthy. As a result, dieting has become big business. Diet magazines enjoy huge circulations. There is almost always a diet book in the best-seller lists. Slimming clubs have thousands of members countrywide. On TV, radio and through newspapers and magazines, there seems to be a never-ending supply of 'new' diets, all promising to achieve what the last one failed to do.

The inadequacy of dieting as a method of weight loss is well known. Many sources estimate that as many as 95% of all people who lose weight by dieting alone regain weight once the diet is over. Yet few 'wonder diet' methods admit this fact. Instead, when a diet fails slimmers are chastised for lack of willpower and greed. Often the fault lies not with the dieter, but with the nature of the diet itself.

WHY DIETS DON'T WORK

Most diets are based on the assumption that the body's only reaction to a smaller intake in food is a drop in weight. False: if food is suddenly and drastically reduced, as happens on a diet, the body reacts by slowing down the rate at which it uses calories, the **basal metabolic rate**.

Why does this happen? Our bodies are programmed for survival, and although the mind may be aware that a diet has started, the body reacts as it would to a period of enforced starvation. It slows the metabolic rate in order to conserve as many calories as possible. As a result, the slimmer who maintained weight on 2,000 calories before dieting, will now find that that amount causes a weight gain.

Crash diets

The worst of all are diets which promise very rapid weight loss. It takes a deficit of about 3,500 calories to lose one pound of fat. The average daily intake for the normally active man is 2,900, the normally active woman 2,100. (Women burn less calories because they are smaller, and have less muscle than men.) A weight-reducing diet generally cuts calorie intake to about 1,000 calories per day for women, 1,800 for men, resulting in a deficit of 1,100 calories daily. It should therefore take at least 3 days to accumulate the deficit of 3,500 necessary to lose one pound.

However, if you have ever started a crash diet, you will know that you can lose more weight than this, often as much as 6lbs in the first three days. How can this be done? The diet is a cheat, a con. You are made to think that the weight you have lost is fat: it isn't. *It is simply water*. And this water will replace itself automatically once the diet is over.

To understand this, the body's reaction to different types of food must be examined. Most rapid weight loss diets are high in protein, and low in carbohydrate. Water in the body attaches itself to a substance called glycogen, and the level of glycogen in the body is controlled by carbohydrate intake.

Thus, when carbohydrate intake is drastically reduced, as happens on a crash diet, glycogen stores are reduced, and the amount of fluid in the body is reduced. This registers as a weight loss on the scales, but it is weight that will be regained immediately once a normal carbohydrate intake is re-established. It is not a fat loss at all.

If a strict diet like this is prolonged, some body fat will be lost, but lean tissue will also be lost from the vital organs (which can be dangerous), and from muscles. The more severe the diet, the more lean tissue is lost. Weight regained after the diet, however, will be fat tissue, so the body will be flabbier and look fatter than previously. And fat tissue is 'lazier' than lean tissue, using less calories, so the dieter is more likely to gain weight than before the diet began. It will also be more difficult to lose weight at the next attempt.

These facts are well known to the medical profession, and have been widely available for years, yet they are scarcely mentioned in any diet book. Instead, these books often issue strict warnings about determination and lack of willpower, making dieters feel guilty and ashamed if they break their diet.

Yet sticking to these programmes requires almost superhuman willpower, because depleted glycogen stores cause intense feelings of hunger. It's like pulling against a spring: your body urges you to eat,

Mastering your diet and nutrition

but your mind insists you can't. If you don't break the diet, you are likely to overeat when you reach target weight, and are freed from the diet. But even if you don't overeat, you will regain weight anyway, because of the greater proportion of lazy fat tissue in your body, because your metabolism has slowed, and because lost fluid will replace itself.

Diet/binge syndrome

Crash dieting is an uphill struggle, therefore, with the body resisting all attempts to shed that weight. Many people, particularly women, have been dieting on and off for years, and the cumulative result is that they now eat a lot less than they did years ago, but they weigh a lot more. Their metabolic rate drops from one diet to the next, making them ever more likely to gain weight.

The psychological effects are devastating. They feel helpless and inadequate because they cannot cope with their problem. They are full of shame, self loathing and self disgust. Their lives are a continual circle of diets, broken by binges when the diets become too much for them.

How can this destructive diet/binge cycle be broken? The answer lies in a regular well-balanced diet, augmented by some form of aerobic exercise. Of course, the dieters have heard that before. And it is advice that they always reject. Your mind is probably jumping in right now saying 'That takes too long, I need something fast', 'What's a balanced diet anyway?' or 'I hate exercise'. The invitation to 'Lose 10lbs in two weeks' sounds much more attractive, so you opt for that yet again.

Permanent weight loss

But before you reject the idea of a sensible eating plan combined with exercise, think of how long you have been trying to lose weight, and the number of times you have tried to diet. (Remember all those wonderful Mondays?)

- **A balanced eating plan, combined with aerobic exercise is guaranteed to give a slow, steady weight loss.** As you lose the weight you will slowly modify your eating and exercising habits, changing the behaviour which made you overweight in the first place.

This is the *only* way to lose weight on a permanent basis. Isn't it worth a try?

Essential nutrients

Nutrient	Function	Food sources
Protein 4 calories per gram	Builds tissue, so essential for growth.	Fish, meat, poultry, eggs, dairy produce, peas, beans, lentils, nuts.
Carbohydrate 4 calories per gram	Essential for metabolic processes.	Cereals and cereal products like bread, other grains eg rice, fruit, vegetables.
Fat 9 calories per gram	Concentrated energy source, insulation.	Fat meat, dairy products, oils, margarine, nuts and seeds, cakes, biscuits.
Fibre	Prevents constipation and related illnesses.	Whole cereal grains, fruit, vegetables, wholemeal bread, pulses and seeds.
Vitamins Vitamin A	Growth of cells, healthy eyesight.	Liver, butter, carrots, margarine, dark green leafy vegetables.
Vitamin B	Good metabolism, healthy nervous system.	Liver, cereals, nuts, fish, meat, vegetables, dairy produce, eggs, poultry.
Vitamin C	Healing of wounds, bones. Aids iron absorption. Keeps body tissue healthy.	Citrus fruits, potatoes, green vegetables, tomatoes, strawberries, blackcurrants.

Fig 50 continued

Vitamin D	Healthy teeth and bones.	Cheese, milk, oily fish, eggs, butter, margarine.
Minerals		
Calcium	Formation of teeth and bones.	Dairy produce, sardines and salmon (with bones), cereals, pulses, green leafy vegetables, nuts and seeds.
Iron	Formation of haemoglobin.	Organ meat, ie liver, kidney, heart, pulses; also cocoa
Zinc	Metabolic processes.	Meat, nuts, peas, wholemeal bread.
Magnesium	Metabolic processes.	Whole grains, green leafy vegetables, soya beans, nuts.

Fig 50: Essential nutrients

A BALANCED DIET

Let's look more closely at the concept of a balanced diet. Most foods, with the exception of alcohol and sugar, contain **nutrients**. Each nutrient has a different function, and they work in combination to maintain a healthy body. Fig 53 describes the most important nutrients, their functions and their main food sources.

In the past, people's diets were unbalanced because they couldn't afford enough protein, or couldn't obtain the fresh food which provides minerals and vitamins. Today, our diets have become unbalanced in a different way. We are eating too much of the wrong types of food.

These are only the *main* nutrients in food. There are many others, some of which probably have not yet been identified. Eating a wide variety of foods will ensure an adequate intake of all nutrients.

The report by the National Advisory Council for Nutritional Education (NACNE) issued in 1983, is generally regarded as the 'bible' of where we are going wrong in our eating habits, and of how to correct the imbalances in the average British diet. Its conclusions can be broadly summarised in four recommendations:

- eat less fat
- eat less sugar
- eat less salt
- eat more fibre

Fat
A diet containing an excess of fat, particularly saturated fat, has been closely linked with death through coronary heart disease. **Saturated fats** are generally of animal origin, meat and dairy products; when reducing fat in the diet, it is mainly this type of fat that should go. But all fat, whether saturated or unsaturated, is extremely high in calories (4 calories per gram protein and carbohydrate, 9 calories per gram fat). So, if weight loss is your aim, it makes sense to cut the fat foods first.

Sugar
Sugar is a substance which is packed with calories, but with nothing else. There are no nutrients in sugar, whether it is white sugar, or brown, or even honey. This also applies to sugar products like sweets and chocolate. They contribute nothing to your diet, except calories, and should be eliminated as much as possible if you are trying to lose weight.

Sugar also makes a significant contribution to tooth decay, and is thought to interfere harmfully with blood sugar levels.

Salt
A diet which is too high in **sodium** (salt) can raise blood pressure, and low-sodium diets have been successful in lowering raised blood pressure for many people. High blood pressure itself has no outward symptoms, but can be a contributing cause to sudden illnesses like heart attacks, or strokes. Our main source of sodium is ordinary table salt, but it is found in many processed, canned and packet foods. Sodium also contributes to **fluid retention**, that unpleasant 'bloated' feeling that most women experience at different stages of the menstrual cycle.

Mastering your diet and nutrition

Fibre

Because fibre isn't absorbed by the body but is excreted, doctors presumed for years that it had no nutritional value. Now a range of diseases, from irritable bowel, diverticulitis, cancer of the bowel, haemorrhoids, and others are being attributed to a lack of fibre in the diet. Fibre absorbs water, provides the bowels with bulk, and smooths the flow of food residue through the system so that there is no strain on the bowels. Fibre foods are also the key to slimness. **Wholegrain** cereals, pulses, vegetables, fruit and nuts provide many essential nutrients, without concentrated amounts of calories.

When preparing food

- Always cut the visible fat from meat.
- Avoid frying food; if you must, use as little oil as possible and ensure that it is a polyunsaturated oil.
- Never fry meat or vegetables before stewing or casseroling.
- Use wholemeal bread, wholewheat pasta and brown rice rather than the white refined versions.
- Avoid using salt at table or in cooking. Instead, take advantage of the large range of herbs and spices for flavouring food.
- Use fresh fruit as dessert, and avoid rich puddings, sweets chocolate, biscuits and cakes as a rule.

THE FOOD GROUPS

Advice like 'Eat more fibre', 'Cut down on fat' or 'Eat a balanced diet' is very vague. It is helpful to divide the various types of nourishing foods that are available to us into four groups:

1. **The milk group** includes milk itself and milk products, like cheese and yoghurt. These foods are a good source of protein, and the main source of calcium in the British diet.

2. **The meat group** is a large group including all kinds of meat, as well as other protein foods like pulses, nuts and fish. Most British people have a sufficient intake of protein.

3. **The fruit and vegetable group** is often neglected, however, and it is the main source of vitamins and minerals.

4. **The cereal group** includes all grains like oats, wheat and rice, plus the bread, breakfast cereals, and pasta products made from them. The unrefined versions of these products are an important source of dietary fibre.

Typical servings from each group:

Protein	Fruit and vegetables	Cereal	Milk
2oz cooked meat or poultry	Piece (uncooked)	Slice bread	Glass milk
3oz fish	4 tbsp cooked	Bowl cereal	Carton yoghurt
2 eggs	Medium serving	3 tbsp rice	1oz cheese
2oz cheese*	Small glass of juice	3 tbsp pasta	
4 tbsp peas, beans or lentils		1 potato	

*(Count cheese as a serving of meat or milk, not both simultaneously.)

Recommended daily servings from each group:

	Protein	Fruit and vegetables	Cereal	Milk
Adult	2	4	4	2
Child	2	4	4	3
Teenager	2	4	4	4
Pregnant woman	3	4	4	4
Nursing mother	2	4	4	4

Fig. 51: The food groups

Mastering your diet and nutrition

Fig 51 outlines typical servings of the foods from each group and the recommended number of servings from each that different people should eat.

The servings are based on the amount of major nutrients present in the different foods, and represent an adequate intake of all essential nutrients. Anybody trying to lose weight will fulfil all their nutritional requirements by sticking to the recommended allowances, and slimmers should try not to go under these allowances.

Physically active people may need more calories than this plan provides; they can add snacks or larger servings once they have included the correct balance from each group.

By using the guidance of the food groups it is possible to devise your own menus so that you take in all the nourishment that your body needs to perform at optimum level without exceeding a reasonable limit of calories. This should eliminate the need for calorie counting.

Vitamins and minerals

There has been a great deal of controversy over the years about the benefits, or otherwise, of taking vitamin and mineral supplements. In the US, more than one third of the population take a vitamin supplement daily. In true American fashion, they have devised the mega-vitamin pill, pills which contain many times the recommended dose. The theory is that if an adequate dose of a vitamin makes you feel good, then large doses should make you feel even better.

The human body does not work like this. Excess doses of vitamin A can cause hair loss, headaches, peeling and itching skin, and in extreme cases enlargement of the liver. Similarly, too much vitamin D can lead to extreme thirst, nausea, kidney failure and deposits of calcium in unsuitable places in the body.

A and D are the only known vitamins that are stored by the body. Surpluses of other vitamins are simply excreted.

Despite this, the British spend millions of pounds on vitamin supplements each year, and the amount continues to grow. The trend towards larger and larger doses of vitamins is also increasing.

Eating sensibly is the most desirable, and the cheapest, method of obtaining your vitamins. As new vitamins and minerals are being discovered all the time, a supplement cannot really compensate for an inadequate diet. A well-balanced intake of food supplies all the body's nutritional needs, including vitamins and minerals.

MAGIC DIET CURE-ALLS

A huge slimming industry has grown up to 'help' those who want to lose weight. If it promises a speedy weight loss, then you name it, somebody has thought of it — starch blockers and appetite suppressants, pills and powders, even jaw wiring and surgery.

Unfortunately, most of these methods do not work. Some can even be dangerous. Slimming has become a hard sell business, invaded by get-rich-quick merchants who are only interested in making money.

Slimming pills

Slimming pills are frowned upon by the medical establishment but they are still sometimes prescribed to dieters. The more common ones include:

- **Appetite suppressants** eg diethylpropion. A survey carried out by the Consumer Association in Britain showed that these products fail to work with the vast majority of slimmers.
- **Thyroid extract** tablets. These speed up the rate at which the body absorbs food. They are dangerous.
- **Diuretics**. These rapidly remove fluid from the body but do nothing to dislodge fat.
- **Starch blockers**. Now banned in the US, with experts agreeing that they are ineffective. Ten million sold in the States before the ban.

Very low calorie diets

One weight loss method which has raised a lot of questions is the Very Low Calorie Diet (VLCD). These are meal replacements — soups, muesli, drinks or bars — which supply all known nutritional needs but a very small number of calories (around 110 for each meal).

The British COMA (Commission on Medical Aspects of Food Policy) Report laid down safety guidelines for such diets. It recommended that no diet should provide less than 40gm of protein for a woman and 50gm for a man. Calorie levels should not fall below 400 per day, and a diet should contain all the required nutrients in one package. Many VLCD companies have introduced new products to bring their diets in line with these recommendations.

Some of the problems associated with VLCDs arise because of the method of distribution. The products are sold by a network of counsellors or advisors who have successfully used the diet themselves. These people are not required to have any medical or nutritional qualifications, and are basically interested in promoting a product. While some counsellors may give excellent back-up and advice, there is the danger that others may be more concerned with making a sale.

In addition, there are doubts as to whether these diets really work. Many dieticians feel that the very selling point of these diets — speedy weight loss — poses problems. As we have seen, losing weight suddenly strips the body of lean tissue as well as fat. When normal eating is resumed the weight tends to return in the form of fat only. This fat tissue uses less calories. Also, if food suddenly becomes short, the body slows the metabolic rate, so that less calories are used for day-to-day living. For both these reasons, a dieter is more prone to gaining weight after a VLCD than they were before they started it.

A third problem is that these diets do nothing to remedy the diet and lifestyle habits that led to a weight problem in the first place. This is essential if weight loss is to be maintained. Nobody can stay on a VLCD forever.

LOSING WEIGHT WITHOUT DIETING

The only type of eating plan you will be able to maintain permanently is one which slightly modifies your existing eating habits. Everybody has different tastes, favourite times of the day for eating, different calorie requirements. Some people hate breakfast, for example; others couldn't survive without it.

To discover your own pattern, keep an **eating diary** for two weeks. In this, record *every* morsel of food, even that single sweet you took from your friend, or the pickings you nibbled while preparing dinner. As a lot of unaccounted calories can be consumed in liquid form — fizzy drinks and alcohol particularly — all drinks should be recorded, too.

If you are a long-term dieter, you may be so used to the diet/binge syndrome that you have no idea what your normal eating pattern is. Put all diets aside for two weeks, and eat exactly what you want, when you want. (If you are a real hardened case, this idea might scare you stiff. Don't panic! You won't balloon to gargantuan proportions in a fortnight. Relax, and plan to enjoy your food thoroughly for once. Just remember to write it all down.)

Your diary should include the time of day that you ate, whether it was a meal or a snack, rough estimates of the amounts of food consumed, and your feelings while eating. Fig 52 gives some examples. Use fig 53 on p.105 to fill in your own eating pattern.

Once you have completed two weeks, examine the pattern and see where you can make cuts, or painless substitutions using the NACNE recommendations. Pay particular attention to cutting fats and sugar, as they are the most important in terms of weight loss.

Remember there is no such thing as a good or bad food. If you adore butter on your bread, then have butter on your bread, but try to cut down on fat in other ways. It is the *balance* of your intake that counts. See how your eating pattern fits into the food groups. Do you tend to eat too much from one group, not enough from another? Many British people eat too much dairy produce, for example, and not enough fruit and vegetables.

Name_____ Date _____

Time(hrs)	*Meal/snack*	*Food eaten*	*Amount*	*Feelings*
0800	Breakfast	Cornflakes, milk and sugar	Large bowl	Hungry.
		Toast, butter and honey	2 slices	
		Coffee (m & s)	1 cup	
1100	Snack	Mars Bar	1	Fed-up, ate to cheer myself up.
		Coffee (m & s)	1 cup	
1300	Lunch	Salad		Not really hungry, ate because it was lunchtime
		Sandwiches	2	
		Soup	1 bowl	
		Coffee (m & s)	1 cup	
		Yoghurt	1 tub	
1530	Snack	Black forest gateau	1 slice	Julie's birthday, ate to be sociable.
		Coffee (m & s)	1 cup	

Fig 52: Example of eating diary

Your eating diary has two uses. Firstly, it shows where you waste calories; for example that extra slice of toast in the mornings eaten out of habit, sugar in your tea that you could do without, those peanuts that you nibble with a drink without even noticing. These are calories that can be cut without effort.

Secondly, your diary will give you an outline of your eating habits, which you can then begin to modify. Remember, your eating pattern is individual to you. By following the NACNE guidelines, and by trying to eat the correct balance from the different food groups, this individual pattern can be modified so that you take in less calories, without subjecting yourself to drastic changes in your eating habits. This is the only pattern you are likely to maintain.

Behaviour modification

Of course, a reduction in food intake and an increase in exercise levels requires discipline. This approach is not going to make things effortless for you. But you won't strain against your body's reactions as you would with a crash low-protein diet, neither will you try to break down ingrained preferences like not eating at night-time.

The secret of behaviour modification is: change what can be changed or what is easy to change, and accept what can't.

Use a low-fat spread and cut down on the amount of spread that you use. Change to low-fat milk. Give up sugar in your tea, if you can do without it, or use an artificial sweetener if you can't. There are lots of improvements that you could make without even noticing.

But if you never eat breakfast and love to eat last thing at night, don't try to change this. Accept it and work around it. Make sure that you have a healthy, low-fat snack to eat around eleven so that you don't choose something that's high in calories. And plan low-calorie suppers for yourself so that you can continue to enjoy your late-night eating without feeling guilty.

Perhaps the opposite is true for you. You couldn't give up butter to save your life. That's fine too. Just make your changes somewhere else that's less painful. Your diary will help you to see what areas are right or wrong for you.

If there is a golden rule, it's this. Don't eat anything unless you are absolutely sure that you want it. Don't eat out of habit, or just because it is teatime. If you are not hungry, or really keen to eat it, don't.

Eating from boredom or frustration is a common problem. The best way to overcome these feelings is to find other ways of coping and exercise can be a good substitute.

This is where discipline — that dreaded word — must come in. Behaviour modification makes things easier because you are not working against your body's natural rhythms and inclinations, but losing weight is never painless. You must exercise regularly in conjunction with your changed eating habits if you are to see a real difference. Similarly, once you have worked out an eating plan from your diary, you must be ruthless about sticking to it.

Although it may be tedious try to maintain your diary throughout this cutting down period, as it keeps you aware of what you are eating.

EATING FOR ACTIVITY

The only group of people more obsessed with diet than slimmers are sportspeople. For centuries, there has been a quest for a miraculous food that would improve athletic ability. Today, most people recognise the importance of good nutrition in achieving peak performance, and that no single 'magic' food can guarantee good nutrition.

The best diet for an exerciser or athlete is very similar to that recommended for everybody else, ie the low-fat, high fibre diet recommended in this chapter.

If you are very active, particularly if you are involved in long distance training, you will probably need a higher calorific intake, as increased exercise means increased expenditure of calories which need to be replaced. The extra calories should take the form of unrefined carbohydrates, that is wholemeal bread and cereals, brown rice, wholewheat pasta, fruit and vegetables, rather than as refined white flour, or sugar products. Refuelling with empty calories leads to vitamin and mineral deficiencies, which will have a detrimental effect on performance.

The traditionally favoured sports diet was the steak-and-cheese-type high protein diet. It was believed that extra protein meant extra muscle and therefore extra strength. It is now recognised that muscle size is determined by the amount of physical demand on it, not by diet, and that excess protein is converted by the body into fat. Carbohydrate is the form of fuel that is most readily available to the body during exercise and so should form the basis of the active person's diet.

Supplementation
A deficiency in vitamin or minerals may take months to show obvious signs, but sporting performance is sure to be affected long before this happens. For this reason, very active people need to monitor their diet constantly to ensure an adequate supply of vitamins and minerals.

Name_____ Date _____

Time(hrs) Meal/snack Food eaten Amount Feelings

0700
0800
0900
1000
1100
1200
1300
1400
1500
1600
1700
1800
1900
2000
2100
2200
2300
2400

Notes

Fig 53: Your eating diary

Indeed, some of these nutrients have functions which are particularly relevant for the sportsperson.

One is iron. Iron is necessary for the formation of haemoglobin in the blood, and as haemoglobin is the substance which carries oxygen around the body, an adequate supply of iron is essential. Liver, heart and kidney, pulses, green leafy vegetables and dried fruits are all good sources of iron. Vitamin C aids its absorption, and because it cannot be stored by the body, vitamin C needs to be taken daily. Good sources are citrus fruits, potatoes, green vegetables and tomatoes.

Folic acid is also essential in the formation of haemoglobin, and in regulating the growth of the cells, including the blood cells. Good sources are liver and kidney, broccoli, spinach, bananas, oranges and pulses.

The simple thing to remember is that these vitamins and minerals and all other essentials are contained in a well-balanced diet as outlined earlier in the chapter. Eat as wide a variety as possible, and be sure to eat enough fruit and vegetables.

8
Planning Your Own Fitness Programme

CONSTRUCTING A PROGRAMME
In Chapter 1, the health-related components of fitness were discussed — aerobic fitness, muscular endurance, muscular strength, flexibility and body composition. All of these components must be developed if your fitness programme is to be balanced.

Constructing a programme that is right for you means analysing each of these components in terms of:

- **Type** — suitable exercises to work on each component.
- **Intensity** — the optimal intensity of exercise to achieve the best results safely.
- **Frequency** — how often each exercise should take place.
- **Duration** — the recommended length of each exercise session.

Exercise to improve aerobic fitness

Type of exercise
Any exercise which causes you to breathe more rapidly and deeply and which raises your heart rate into training zone and keeps it there for some time. The most effective aerobic exercises are rhythmical and repetitive, eg brisk walking, jogging, running, swimming, cycling, aerobic dancing.

Intensity of exercise
60% to 85% of training heart rate (THR). Research increasingly indicates that aerobic exercise does not have to take place at high intensity to be effective.

Duration of exercise
In order to be effective, aerobic exercise must continue for at least twenty minutes at THR.

Frequency of exercise session
Three times per week at equally spaced intervals.

Exercise to improve muscular endurance

Type of exercise
Any exercise which requires a muscle or muscle group to perform a movement repeatedly. Resistance training is most effective.

Intensity of exercise
Low. Because the action must be performed repeatedly, resistance cannot be high. Intensity should be low enough to allow you to perform at least 25 repetitions of the exercise with good technique.

Duration of exercise
A balanced muscular endurance programme can be completed in forty-five minutes (including warm-up and cool-down). Two or three sets of 25 reps each exercise.

Frequency of exercise session
Three times per week at equally spaced intervals.

Exercise to improve muscular strength

Type of exercise
Any exercise which requires a muscle to exert force against maximal or sub-maximal resistance, ie weight training.

Intensity of exercise
High to very high — the maximum amount of weight that can be lifted for 1 to 8 reps.

Duration of exercise
While keen strength/body builders spend hours in the gym, the average person can achieve appropriate strength improvements in the major muscle groups in a 45 minute session (including warm-up and cool-down): three sets of 1 to 8 reps of each exercise.

Frequency of exercise session
Four times per week at equally spaced intervals.

Exercise to improve flexibility

Type of exercise
Any exercise which takes muscles and joints beyond their normal range of movement, ie stretching.

Planning your own fitness programme

Intensity of exercise
Stretching exercises are difficult to describe in terms of intensity. You should feel that you have stretched as far as possible without experiencing pain.

Duration of exercise
Each position needs to be held for approximately thirty seconds. A good stretch session covering the major muscle groups can be achieved in fifteen minutes.

Frequency of exercise
Three times per week at equally spaced intervals.

Exercise to improve body composition (less body fat)

Type of exercise
Aerobic exercise such as brisk walking, jogging, running, cycling, swimming, aerobic dancing.

Intensity of exercise
Low intensity. 60% to 75% of THR.

Duration of exercise
At least thirty minutes

Frequency of exercise
Four times per week at regularly spaced intervals.

EXAMPLE PROGRAMME

Let us take an example. Anne is a 35-year-old executive, in good health. But she has not exercised since she left school, and is leading a sedentary lifestyle, travelling to work by car and sitting at her desk all day.

She is concerned about her weight (or more accurately her body composition) and also about the fact that she is out of breath if she climbs one flight of stairs. She wants to shape up, lose some fat, become fitter.

A walk/jog programme will help Anne to achieve many of her aims. Because it is so long since she exercised she must begin very slowly (see Chapter 3). Once she is in a position to walk/jog at THR for a continuous minimum of thirty minutes, four times per week, she should lose body fat and greatly improve her aerobic fitness.

This activity will also improve the muscular strength/endurance of Anne's lower body; this improvement will need to be balanced by a resistance training programme for the upper body. She will also need to do stretching exercises to improve her flexibility.

Strength/endurance and stretching exercises should be done three times per week for maximum benefits. She can do them on the same day as her walk/jog session, or on alternate days. Fifteen minutes for each should be ample.

So Anne's programme looks like this?
- **walk/jog** — four times per week for continuous 30 minutes (plus).
- **stretch** — three times per week for 15 minutes.
- **endurance** exercises (upper body) — 3 sets of 20 to 25 reps, three times per week for about 15 minutes.

For an input of about four hours per week Anne should achieve all her fitness and figure aims.

YOUR EXERCISE PROGRAMME

With reference to the above guidelines, you can now devise your own exercise programme. Ask yourself the following questions:

- What benefits do I intend to get from this programme?
- Which fitness components am I most interested in improving?
- Which limiting factors (age, medical background and so on) do I need to take into account?

The questionnaires and charts which you have filled out while reading this book will help you to answer these questions in more details. The **lifestyle questionnaire** (page 22) will help you to analyse your current lifestyle and pinpoint areas which may be causing problems for you, while the **fitness assessment chart** (page 19) will rate your score in each of the health-related components of fitness. Your **eating diary** (page 105) will help you to assess your current eating habits and show where improvements can be made.

Armed with this information, you are ready to devise your exercise programme. Aerobic exercise, strength/endurance and flexibility charts are provided to allow you to record the type, intensity, duration and frequency of each type of exercise. (Photocopy the charts as you will need to use them again and again.)

As you fill out these charts over the weeks, you will find that the intensity and the duration of your workouts increase. This is a clear sign of your improvement: your body is capable of efforts which were beyond it a few short weeks before.

Improvement can also be recorded by regularly re-assessing your performance on the fitness test outlined in Chapter 1. You should re-do these tests every twelve weeks or so (re-assessment more often than this is not advisable, as improvements are unlikely to be significant.)

Aerobic exercise chart

Week ending_____   Resting heart rate _____

         Date   *Activity*   *Duration*   *Comments*
Session 1 _____
Session 2 _____
Session 3 _____
Session 4 _____

Week ending_____   Resting heart rate _____

         Date   *Activity*   *Duration*   *Comments*
Session 1 _____
Session 2 _____
Session 3 _____
Session 4 _____

Week ending_____   Resting heart rate _____

         Date   *Activity*   *Duration*   *Comments*
Session 1 _____
Session 2 _____
Session 3 _____
Session 4 _____

Week ending_____   Resting heart rate _____

         Date   *Activity*   *Duration*   *Comments*
Session 1 _____
Session 2 _____
Session 3 _____
Session 4 _____

Fig. 54: Aerobic exercise chart

Strength/endurance chart

Week ending _____

	Session 1 W R S	Session 2 W R S	Session 3 W R S
Squats			
Leg raises			
Heel raise			
Kneeling kick back			
Side leg lifts			
Bench press			
Bench flyes			
Arm curl			
Tricep press			
Shoulder press behind neck			
Upright rowing			
Lateral raises			
Spinal hyperextension			
Abdominal curl up			
Reverse abdominal curl			
Diagonal crunch			
Pelvic floor lifts			

W = weight
R = reps
S = sets   *Time* =

Fig. 55: Strength/endurance chart

Planning your own fitness programme

Flexibility chart

Week ending _____

	Session 1	Session 2	Session 3
Gastrocnemius stretch			
Soleus stretch			
Quadriceps stretch			
Hip flexor stretch			
Hamstring stretch			
Gluteal stretch			
Abductor stretch			
Adductor stretch			
Erector spinae (lower back) stretch			
Rectus abdominus stretch			
Erector spinae (upper back) stretch			
Posterior deltoid and trapezius stretch			
Biceps, anterior deltoid and pectoral stretch			
Triceps stretch			
Neck stretches			
Time:			

Fig. 56: Flexibility chart

SPECIAL CONSIDERATIONS

Age

Most fitness characteristics decrease with age. If a group of 'average' people from 20 to 80 years are tested and the results plotted, a steady deterioration occurs with each decade. This decline, starting in the middle 20s, has been called the **aging curve**.

However, a portion of the deterioration seen in aging curves is caused by less activity in older individuals — not by aging itself. People who maintain active lifestyles have a slower fitness decline than is seen in typical aging curves.

Age must be taken into consideration when devising fitness programmes. In the elderly population, maintaining bone mineral content and flexibility in the limbs is increasingly important, along with a reasonable level of aerobic fitness. Controlled fitness activities are best, rather than vigorous sports which might be too intense and where deterioration in skills like agility or reaction time might cause safety problems.

At the other end of the age scale, the opposite applies. Games, sports and fun activities are more appropriate for the under-twenties than specific fitness programmes. Intensive strength training is particularly unsuitable for young unformed bones and muscles.

Pregnancy

For the first third of pregnancy the baby's life support system, the placenta, is being manufactured. Throughout the nine months the mother's heart, lungs and other vital organs are working much harder than usual. Hormonal changes make joints less stable, and unaccustomed posture and loose ligaments can lead to clumsiness.

So, no matter how fit you are, now matter how accustomed to exercise, pregnancy brings changes in physiology and anatomy which must be considered while exercising.

Pregnancy introduces new exercise objectives — exercising to lose weight or improve fitness is not appropriate. Rather, the objectives of an exercise programme should be:

- To improve posture, both standing and moving posture, during exercise and on a daily basis.
- To maintain general mobility.
- To promote the circulation throughout the body, especially in the feet and ankles.
- To strengthen the pelvic floor and other relevant muscle groups.
- To improve neuromuscular control, aiding relaxation of specific

Planning your own fitness programme

body parts. As you will learn in any pre-natal exercise class, this is an important part of coping with the pain of labour.
- To improve body awareness and maintain a good self image during pregnancy.

So this is *not* the time to start a get-fit programme or to try to lose weight! If you are unused to exercise, the only activity you should contemplate before the baby is born is specific ante-natal classes. Your doctor should have details.

If you are a regular exerciser, there is no reason why you should not continue your normal exercise programme, with your doctor's permission. However, because of the changes which take place in pregnancy, you may need to modify your programme slightly. For example, your pulse rate should not rise above approximately 140 beats per minute during aerobic exercise.

Hormonal changes must also be taken into account. The release of **relaxin** is one of the chief of these in pregnancy. The hormone is well named — it causes the ligaments to relax so the pelvis can widen and accommodate the baby during pregnancy and childbirth. This effect is general to the whole body, not specific to the pelvis; the slackening of ligaments affects the stability of all joints in the body.

Experts fear that stretching ligaments and muscles to their limits during pregnancy may cause problems. Because of the presence of relaxin, ligaments may become overstretched, causing permanent problems with joint stability.

Relaxed ligaments can also cause discomfort in the pelvic region. The big bones of the pelvis are joined in the front by the pubis symphysis, a normally immovable joint in the pubic bones in front, and at the back by the sacro-iliac joint at the base of the spine. Relaxed ligaments mean that these joints are less stable than usual. Movements in these areas — particularly wide open legged stretches — may cause discomfort, even pain.

Another potential problem is the use of exercises to strengthen abdominal muscles, for example the sit-up. The rectus abdominus — a broad band of muscle running down the front of the body — separates during pregnancy to allow the uterus to expand as the baby grows. Once separation of the rectus abdominus has occurred, abdominal exercises against resistance, like the sit-up, can cause a pull in an unusual direction. This exaggerates the separation, and there is a danger that an enlarged tummy will not return to normal after the birth. Bear in mind, too, that a pregnant woman should not lie on her back for lengthy periods of time after four months, as the weight of the growing foetus could compress a blood vessel, inhibiting circulation.

Be careful about attending classes or health clubs during pregnancy. Many otherwise qualified teachers are not *au fait* with pre- or postnatal exercise. Do not take chances with your body (and your baby) if you have doubts.

MAINTAINING A FIT LIFESTYLE

The first weeks of an exercise programme will reward you with the most rapid results. In the first twelve weeks aerobic fitness typically improves by 15% - 25%. Strength and endurance improvements will be marked, too. It is not unusual to be able to lift twice as much weight, twice as often, after only twelve weeks of regular strength/endurance training.

Flexibility will be greatly improved. If a balanced exercise programme is combined with a balanced diet of lower calorific intake, body composition should also be vastly improved. All exercise adaptations occur more rapidly in those people who have never exercised before.

But the fitter you become, the smaller the measurable changes. Typically, the changes which take place between week 1 and week 12 of an exercise programme are more marked than those which occur between week 12 and week 24. This is to be expected and should not cause disappointment.

Eventually you will reach a stage where you are happy with the new, fit, slim you. To maintain this level of fitness and shape is relatively easy. As long as you continue to exercise as the same intensity for the same length of time, one or two sessions per week should be enough to maintain your condition.

You may find, however, that you continue to exercise more often than this, just for the enjoyment of it. Exercise is not just about being fitter and healthier: it is also a physical pleasure, a deeply satisfying pleasure which cannot be appreciated by the sedentary.

The joy of running, light and free in the fresh air, on a crisp winter morning; the glow of muscles which have been put through a vigorous workout; the fun of moving in unison with twenty others in time to music; the feeling of energy, control, get-up-and-go which goes hand in hand with being fit: these pleasures, and so many others, are marvellous reasons for exercising regularly.

Our bodies were made to move, and when we exercise, we are rewarded in all sorts of ways. These rewards are yours for the taking. Enjoy yourself!

Glossary

Aerobic exercise. Any repetitive, rhythmical exercise involving the large muscle groups of the body so that the heart rate is raised into the training zone and maintained there for a continuous minimum of twenty to thirty minutes. Good examples are running, cycling, swimming, dancing.

Aerobic fitness. Ability of cardiovascular system to provide oxygen for exercising muscles as above.

Artery. A blood vessel carrying blood from the heart to body tissues.

Atherosclerosis. A disease in which the inner layer of the artery wall becomes thick and irregular with deposits of fatty substances.

Agonist. A muscle directly engaged in contraction.

Antagonist. Opposing muscle to agonist.

Arthritis. Inflammation of a joint.

Ballistic exercise. Bouncing movements which can stress joints and muscles.

Blood pressure. The pressure exerted by the blood on the vessel walls.

Body composition. The relative amounts of muscle, bone and fat in the body. Usually divided into fatness (% body fat) and leanness (% lean body mass).

Calorie. Amount of heat required to raise the temperature of 1g of water by 1 degree celsius. Used as a measure of energy (provided by food and used by activity).

Cardiorespiratory endurance (CRE). Fitness of the cardiovascular and respiratory systems. See **Aerobic fitness.**

Cardiovascular system. The heart and blood vessels and circulation of the blood through them.

Contraindicated exercise. An exercise which is medically inadvisable for a particular individual.

Coronary arteries. Blood vessels supplying the heart muscle.

Coronary heart disease (CHD). See **Atherosclerosis**.

Duration. Length of time for a fitness workout.

Exercise modification. Adjustment of exercise programme in terms of type of activity, intensity, frequency and duration to match exerciser's physical condition and fitness objectives.

Exercise progression. The increase in total work and/or intensity as the exerciser progresses from sedentary lifestyle to state of fitness.

Fartlek. A formal method of training, also known as speed play, which alternates fast and slow running over varied terrain.

Fitness assessment. Evaluation and measurement of the various components of fitness. Fitness assessments can vary from simple home tests which can give only a general indication of fitness to scientific evaluations under laboratory conditions.

Flexibility. The ability to move the joints through their full range of motion without discomfort.

Frequency. How often a person has a fitness workout.

Haemoglobin. The pigment in the red blood corpuscles which carries oxygen.

Health-related components of fitness. Those aspects of fitness pertaining to health: aerobic fitness, muscular strength, muscular endurance, flexibility, body composition.

Heart rate. The number of beats of the heart per minute.

Hypertension. High blood pressure — blood pressure in excess of normal values for age and gender.

Intensity. The magnitude of energy required for a particular activity.

Interval training. A training system which alternates harder and lighter work.

Inverse stretch reflex. A reflex action brought into play when a muscle is stretched to its full extent and held there for 6 seconds or more. The antagonist muscle to that being stretched relaxes, allowing the muscle to be further stretched without damage.

Isometric exercise. A static muscle contraction, with no movement of body parts. Muscle length does not change.

Glossary

Isotonic exercise. Exercise which develops muscle through a full range of movement, involving shortening or lengthening of the muscle.

Joint. Where two bones join.

Long slow distance training. Also called 'continuous training.' Activity of low/medium intensity maintained for relatively long periods, such as brisk walking, jogging, leisurely cycling. This type of exercise is most effective in reducing body fat levels.

Maximum heart rate (MHR). The highest heart rate attainable. A person's maximum heart rate can be estimated by subtracting age from 220.

Metabolic rate. Rate at which energy is consumed, ie calories used.

Metabolism. The process of chemical changes by which energy is provided for the maintenance of life.

Mobility exercises. Exercises to mobilise the joints.

Muscular endurance. The ability of a muscle to exert a force repeatedly over a period of time — a long-term activity at less than maximum effort.

Muscular strength. The maximum amount of force which can be exerted by a muscle — an all out, short-term effort.

Nerve spindles. Nerve endings whose main function is to send messages to the brain from the muscles, giving information about the state of stretch.

Obesity. Storage of excess body fat. Obese people have an increased risk of developing CHD, diabetes and hypertension.

Overload. To place greater than usual demands upon the body.

Pulse raiser. Exercise which makes the heart beat more quickly, thereby increasing the flow of blood to the working muscles and raising the body temperature in preparation for activity to come.

Resistance. The amount of force applied opposite a movement.

Respiration. The act or function of breathing.

Resting Heart Rate (RHR). The number of times the heart beats per minute when the body is at rest. Best taken before getting out of bed in the morning.

Glossary

Spot reducing. Trying to lose fat at one body site doing exercises centred on that site. No research evidence supports this concept.

Stretching. Extending the limbs through a full range of motion.

Stretch reflex. A protective reflex to overstretching or ballistic movements which causes the muscle to contract.

Training heart rate (THR). The rate at which an exerciser's heart should beat during a fitness workout in order to achieve training benefits.

Vitamin. An organic substance that is present in small amounts in food and that is necessary for the normal functioning of the cells.

Useful Addresses

Alcohol Concern, 305 Gray's Inn Road, London WC1X 8QF (071-833 3471).

Amateur Athletic Association, Francis House, Francis Street, London SW1P 1DL (071-828 9326).

ASH, Action on Smoking and Health, 5/11 Mortimer Street, London W1N 7RJ (071-637 9843).

ASSET, The National Association for Health and Exercise Teachers, 112a Great Russell Street, London WC1B 3NQ (071-580 4451).

British Cycling Federation, 16 Upper Woburn Place, London WC1H 0PQ (071-387 9320).

British Heart Foundation, 102 Gloucester Place, London W1H 4DH (071-935 6185).

British Nutrition Foundation, 15 Belgrave Square, London SW1X 8PS (071-235 4904).

British Red Cross Society, 9 Grosvenor Crescent, London SW1X 7EJ (071-235 5454).

British Sports Association for the Disabled, Tottenham Sports, Hayward House, Barnard Crescent, Aylesbury, Bucks HP21 8PP (0296- 27889).

Health Education Council, 78 New Oxford Street, London WC1 1AH (071-631 0930).

National Coaching Foundation, 4 College Close, Beckett Park, Leeds LS6 3QH (0532-744802).

Overeaters Anonymous, c/o Manor Garden Centre, 6-9 Manor Gardens, London N7 6JY (081-868 4109).

Physical Education Association, Ling House, 162 King's Cross Road, London WC1X 9DH (071-278 9311).

Royal Life Saving Society, Mountbatten House, Studley, Warwicks BS0 7NN (052-785 3943).

Sports Council, 16 Upper Woburn Place, London WC1H 0PQ (071-388 1277).

St John Ambulance, 1 Grosvenor Crescent, London SW1X 7EF (071-235 5231).

Women's Sports Foundation, 70 Great Queen Street, London WC2 (071-831 7863).

Further reading

Anderson, Bob, *Stretching*, Pelham (1980).

Binney, R., ed., *The BUPA Manual of Fitness and Wellbeing*, Macdonald & Co (1984).

Cannon, G. and Eising, H., *Dieting Makes You Fat*.

Collum R. and Mowbray L., *The English YMCA Guide to Exercise to Music*, Pelham (1986).

Cooper K. H., *The New Aerobics*, Bantam (1970).

East, R. and Towers, B., *No Smoke*, Kingston Polytechnic (1979). (Available from Botes Books, Brook Street, Kingston-upon-Thames or by order from your local bookshop.)

Grisogono V., *Sports Injuries: A Self Help Guide*, John Murray (1984).

Grant, M. and Gwinner P., *What's Your Poison?*, BBC (1979).

Maryon-Davies, A. and Thomas, J., *Diet 2000: How to Eat for A Healthier Future*, Pan (1984).

Prytherch, R., *Sports and Fitness: An Information Guide*, Gower (1988).

Orbach, Susie, *Fat is a Feminist Issue*, Paddington Press (1978).

Payne, Mark, Dr., *How to Take Care of Your Heart*, Northcote House (1989).

Taylor, E., *Progressive Weight Training for Men and Women*, Springfield (1988).

Wilmore, Jack H., *Sensible Fitness*, Illinois: Leisure Press (1986).

Know the Game Series (A&C Black). 70 booklets with basic information relating to the most common sports.

Index

Abdominal curl-up, 62
Abdominal hold, 17
Abdominal muscles, conditioning of, 62–64
Abduction, leg, 30–31, 54–55
Abductor stretch, 74
Abrasion, 85
Adductor stretch, 75
Aerobic exercise, 38–41
Aerobic fitness, 11–12, 17, 35–38
Aerobics class, see exercise class, 45–46
Aging and exercise, 114
Alcohol, 21
Arm curl, 58
Atherosclerosis, 36

Balanced diet, 95
Ballistic stretching, 68–69
Basal metabolic rate, 91
Behaviour modification, 103
Bench flyes, 57
Bench press, 56
Blisters, 86
Blood pressure, see hypertension, 36
Body composition, 14, 36
　effects of exercise, 37
Bone disease, 38
Bursitis, 86

Carbohydrates, 94
Cardiorespiratory endurance, 35–38
Cardiovascular system, disease of, 36, 87
Cigarette smoking, 20–21
Circuits, 49
Contraindicated exercise, 15, 80–83
Contusions, 86

Cool-down phase, 33–34
　for runners, 43–44
Crash diets, 92–93
Cycling, 45

Diagonal crunches, 64
Diet
　crash diets, 92
　dietary aids, 100–101
　diet/binge syndrome, 93
　dietary supplements, 99, 104–106
Dislocations, 86
Double leg raises, 82
Dynamic posture, 29–31

Eating diary, 102
Erector spinae stretch, 75–76
Essential nutrients, 94–95
Exercise,
　body composition and, 36–37
　contraindications to, 15
　screening for, 15
　age and, 114
　nutrition and, 104
　pregnancy and, 114
　safety and, 80–88
Exercise classes, 45–46

Fartlek, 45
Fats, 94, 96
Fibre, 94, 97
First aid, 88
Fitness, benefits of, 9–10
Fitness assessment/testing, 16–19
Fixx, James, 80
Flexibility, 13, 67–78
Food groups, 97–99

Index

Fractures, 86
Frequency of exercise, 41
Front of arm, shoulder, chest stretch, 77

Gastrocnemicus stretch, 71
Gluteal stretch, 74
Gymnasium, choosing a good one, 65–66

Hamstrings stretch, 73
Health screening, 14–15
Health-related components of fitness, 10–14
Heart disease, 36
Heart rates, 39–40
Heel raise, 52–53
High blood pressure, see hypertension, 36
Hip flexor stretch, 72–73
Hypertension, 36

Imbalance injuries, 88
Incisions, 85
Injuries, 85–89
    treatment of minor, 89
Intensity of exercise, 38–40, 107–109
Interval training, 44
Inverse stretch reflex, 69

Jogging, see running, 41–45

Kneeling kick-back, 54

Lacerations, 85
Lateral arm raises, 61
Leg raises, 53
Lifestyle,
    analysis, 22–23
    a healthy lifestyle, 24–24, 116
Lower leg lifts, 55

Maximum heart rate, 39
Measurements, body circumference, 19
Minerals, 94, 99

Mobility exercises, 32–33
Muscle contraction, forms of, 48
Muscle cramps, 83
Muscle injury, 67
Muscle soreness, 50–51
Muscular endurance, 12–13, 50, 51–65
Muscular strength, 12–13, 50, 51–65

Neck stretches, 78

Obesity, 36–37
Overload, principle of, 48
Overuse injuries, 88

Pelvic tilt, 28
Pinch test, 18
Posture, 25–31
Progressive resistance, principle of, 49
Protein, 94
Puncture wounds, 85

Quadriceps stretch, 72–73

Rectus Abdominus stretch, 76
Rehabilitation after injury, 90
Relaxation, 79
Repetitions, 49
Resistance training programme, 49–65
Reverse abdominal curl, 63
Running, 41–45

Safety, 80–90
Salt, 96
Sets, 49
Seated shoulder press behind neck, 25
Seated triceps extension, 58
Shin splints, 86
Side leg raises, 30–31, 54-55
Sit, how to, 26–27
Sit and reach test, 18
Sit-ups, 86

Index

Skill related fitness components, 11
Slimming, 91–104
Sprains, 86
Spinal hyperextension, 62
Spotter, 49
Squats, 52
Stand, how to, 26–27
Static stretch, 69
Straight leg sit ups, 81–82
Strains, 86
Stress, 21
Stretch reflex, 69
Stretching,
    importance of, 67–68
    programme, 70–78
Sugar, 96
Swinging toe touches, 83

Tendonitis, 67, 86
Training heart rate (THR), 39
Training session, duration of, 41
Training systems, 44–45
Traumatic injury, 87
Triceps stretch, 78

Upper back stretch, 77
Upright rowing, 60

Vitamins, 94, 99

Walking, 41
Walk/jog/run programme, 41–42
Warm up, 32–33
    for runners, 44